the

chronic
obstructive
pulmonary
disease

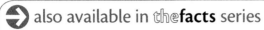 **also available in the facts series**

the**facts**

chronic obstructive pulmonary disease

GRAEME P. CURRIE

OXFORD
UNIVERSITY PRESS

OXFORD

UNIVERSITY PRESS

Great Clarendon Street, Oxford OX2 6DP

Oxford University Press is a department of the University of Oxford.
It furthers the University's objective of excellence in research, scholarship,
and education by publishing worldwide in

Oxford New York

Auckland Cape Town Dar es Salaam Hong Kong Karachi
Kuala Lumpur Madrid Melbourne Mexico City Nairobi
New Delhi Shanghai Taipei Toronto

With offices in

Argentina Austria Brazil Chile Czech Republic France Greece
Guatemala Hungary Italy Japan Poland Portugal Singapore
South Korea Switzerland Thailand Turkey Ukraine Vietnam

Oxford is a registered trade mark of Oxford University Press
in the UK and in certain other countries

Published in the United States
by Oxford University Press Inc., New York

British Library Cataloguing in Publication Data

Data available

Library of Congress Cataloging in Publication Data

Data available

ISBN 978–0–19–956368–5

10 9 8 7 6 5

Typeset in Plantin
by Cepha Imaging Pvt. Ltd., Bangalore, India
Printed in China through
Asia Pacific Offset

Whilst every effort has been made to ensure that the contents of this book are as complete, accurate,
and up-to-date as possible at the date of writing, Oxford University Press is not able to give any
guarantee or assurance that such is the case. Readers are urged to take appropriately qualified
medical advice in all cases. The information in this book is intended to be useful to the general
reader, but should not be used as a means of self-diagnosis or for the prescription of medication.

Printed in Great Britain by Clays Ltd, St Ives plc

Preface

What is chronic obstructive pulmonary disease?

Chronic obstructive pulmonary disease (COPD) is an all too common lung condition, which varies markedly in severity between individuals. COPD is the term that covers conditions previously known as chronic bronchitis and emphysema. It is associated with impaired lung function that fails to change significantly over time. As a result, it causes progressive symptoms such as breathlessness, wheeze, cough, reduced exercise tolerance, and frequent chest infections. In mild disease, patients only have symptoms during exertion; as the condition develops, some of these symptoms may occur at rest. Cigarette smoking is the main cause of COPD, and quitting should underpin its management. Other than with determination and willpower, this can be achieved with the help of counselling, nicotine replacement therapy, and certain drugs. Other strategies in the management of COPD can be divided into non-drug and drug treatment. Non-drug treatment consists of pulmonary rehabilitation, vaccination, dietary input, and education. The main drugs used in its treatment are inhaled short- and long-acting bronchodilators (drugs that open the airways) and inhaled steroids. Other types of drug include theophylline, mucolytics, and steroid tablets. A minority of patients with advanced disease may benefit from long-term oxygen for use on a daily basis at home. Patients may have intermittent worsening of COPD (called an exacerbation). Exacerbations are usually managed at home, although some patients may require admission to hospital. They are usually treated with steroid tablets, antibiotics, and inhaled short-acting bronchodilators to open up the airways. In patients with severe exacerbations, more intensive hospital treatment, using a machine to assist breathing (non-invasive or invasive ventilator), can sometimes be necessary.

Why should I read this book?

It is fairly well known that the more people know about an illness or condition, the less they fear it. Furthermore, the more you understand about your illness the better equipped you are to deal with the problems that arise and this may enable you to work more closely and effectively with doctors and nurses. This book may also provide the carers of someone with COPD a greater understanding of the condition and help them to encourage their relative/spouse/ friend to live with COPD rather than live in fear of it.

Who is this book for?

This book is designed for patients, their carers, all cigarette smokers, and all others interested in COPD; it may also be of some use to professions allied to medicine such as nurses, physiotherapist, and occupational therapists. It provides an easy to read up-to-date account of COPD and its management. The overall aim of the book is to increase the amount of reliable and accessible information, which may help, in some way, to reduce the burden of COPD in the community at large.

Acknowledgements

I would like to thank Aileen Currie, senior pharmacist at Crosshouse Hospital, and staff nurses Menna Forgrieve and Sue Fox of the Chest Clinic at Aberdeen Royal Infirmary for reading and commenting on the text. I would also like to thank Sister Sandra Steele for making suggestions regarding the text and for help with figures.

Contents

1

How the normal lungs work

Key points

♦ Air containing oxygen passes through the mouth and nose into the windpipe (trachea). The windpipe then divides repeatedly into smaller branches of increasingly narrow size (bronchi and bronchioles) within the lungs.

♦ The smallest air passages (bronchioles) end as tiny air sacs (alveoli) where gas exchange takes place; oxygen passes from the air sacs into the blood and carbon dioxide passes from the blood into the air sacs.

♦ The left lung consists of two lobes and the right lung consists of three lobes.

♦ Oxygen is transported throughout the body in red blood cells.

♦ The whole process of transportation of oxygen to the body by way of the heart, arteries, capillaries, veins, and lungs is called the circulation.

♦ The act of breathing is under automatic control by the brain and consists of inspiration and expiration.

Air passages

At rest, most healthy people breathe through the nose, although this may change to the mouth when the nose is blocked (e.g. when you have a 'cold') and when exercising. Atmospheric air (containing 21% oxygen) is inhaled through either the mouth or the nose, and passes into a long tube-like structure called the windpipe (trachea). The windpipe is made up of 'C'-shaped rings of cartilage (which is like soft bone), which you can feel in the midline of

1

the neck; these rings prevent the windpipe from collapsing. It then divides behind the breast bone (sternum) within the chest into two smaller air passages (bronchi), on the left and right sides, which lead into the lungs. These two main bronchi then subdivide even further into smaller branches (called lobar bronchi). These subdivide repeatedly into increasingly smaller branches (called segmental bronchi and bronchioles) and ultimately end in millions of small air sacs (alveoli). It is in these air sacs that a process called gas exchange occurs. This means that oxygen passes from the air sacs into the bloodstream and is then transported around the body. The waste gas carbon dioxide passes from the bloodstream into the air sacs and is eventually exhaled by breathing out through the nose or mouth.

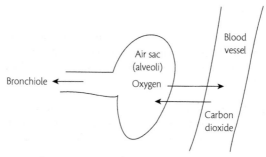

Fig. 1.1 Diagrammatic representation of air sacs (alveoli) and the process of gas exchange.

Lungs

The lungs are two cone-shaped structures lying within the chest cavity. They extend from the neck above to the diaphragm (a thin layer of muscle separating the chest cavity from the abdominal cavity) below. Between each lung is found a variety of important structures such as:

◆   the heart;

◆   major blood vessels (a mixture of large arteries and veins);

◆   lymph glands and lymph vessels;

◆   the windpipe (trachea);

◆   the gullet.

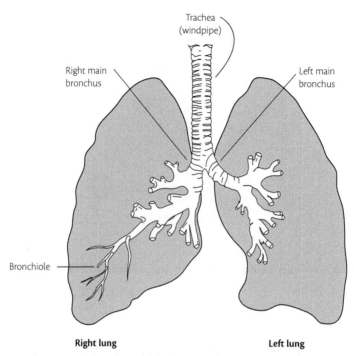

Fig. 1.2 The airway, its branches, and the lungs.

Since the heart lies mainly on the left side of the chest, the right lung is slightly larger than the left lung. The right lung consists of three lobes and the left lung consists of two lobes. The lobes of the lung are made up mainly of millions of air passages (bronchi and bronchioles), air sacs (alveoli), lymph glands and lymph vessels, blood vessels, and surrounding (or connecting) tissues.

The lungs are surrounded by two thin layers called the pleura. The pleura are separated from one another by a small amount of fluid that acts as a lubricant between them. This allows the pleura to slide easily against each other without any friction when the lungs increase and decrease in size during breathing. This fluid is rather like a thin film of water trapped between two layers of glass; the layers can easily slide over one another but cannot be easily pulled apart. The outer layer of pleura is firmly attached to the inside of the chest wall.

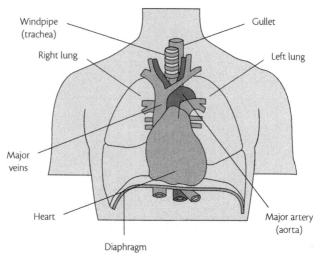

Fig. 1.3 The relationship between the heart, lungs, and other structures found in the chest.

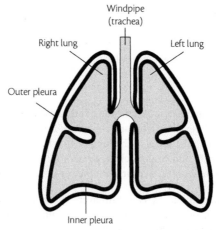

Fig. 1.4 Diagrammatic representation of the lungs and inner and outer pleura.

Breathing

Breathing involves two main actions: inspiration (breathing in) and expiration (breathing out). The action of breathing is largely under the control of the breathing centre of the brain and occurs spontaneously (around 12 breaths per minute in resting healthy adults). However, we all have some control over how fast or slow we breathe and it may alter in response to a variety of triggers such as fear, anxiety, exercise, illness, or pain. When breathing in, muscles of the chest (mainly the diaphragm and muscles between the ribs (intercostal muscles)) cause the lungs to increase in size—you can consider this to be like a partially filled balloon being blown up further. During periods where deeper breathing is necessary (e.g. during exercise), other muscles of the chest and neck help in this process. When breathing out, the diaphragm and intercostal muscles relax and the inflated lungs partially deflate—like some of the air being let out of a filled balloon.

Circulation of blood

Red blood cells, which are one of several constituents of blood, carry oxygen around the body. Blood (containing red blood cells) is pumped throughout the body by vessels called arteries. The main artery of the body, which arises from the left side of the heart, is called the aorta; the aorta subdivides into many other smaller arteries, which supply all the organs and tissues of the body. The various organs and tissues of the body extract oxygen from red blood cells via smaller blood vessels called capillaries and release the waste gas, carbon dioxide. Veins then transport blood (without a supply of oxygen but with carbon dioxide) to the right side of the heart. The two main veins that enter the right side of the heart (and ultimately collect blood from all the veins in the body) are called the superior and inferior vena cava. From the right side of the heart, blood containing red blood cells then passes through both lungs and become enriched with oxygen again. Carbon dioxide is transferred from the bloodstream into the lungs. This whole process of transportation of oxygen

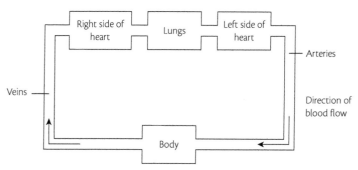

Fig. 1.5 Diagrammatic representation of how blood passes through the heart, arteries, veins, and lungs (the circulation).

to the body, with the help of the heart, arteries, capillaries, veins, and lungs, is called the circulation.

When things go wrong

As described above, nature has developed a highly efficient system by which to keep us all feeling alive and well. This is largely by making sure that all our organs and tissues are supplied with plenty of oxygen and that waste products are removed. When things start to go wrong with parts of this process, we often know about it mainly due to the appearance of:

◆ symptoms—these are things that you feel wrong with you such as breath-lessness, cough, reduced exercise tolerance and wheeze.

◆ signs—these are physical abnormalities that doctors or nurses find when they examine you.

In chronic obstructive pulmonary disease (COPD), it is the lungs that are predominantly affected and your body will usually react to this by making you aware that there might be something going wrong.

2

What is COPD?

⮕ Key points

♦ COPD is a long-term condition that is associated with impaired lung function and lung damage. It usually becomes worse over time if cigarette smoking continues.

♦ It is relatively common and is thought to affect over 1 million individuals in the UK.

♦ COPD is uncommon in people below 35 years of age and most often becomes apparent in those over 65 years of age.

♦ It causes around 5% of all deaths each year in the UK.

♦ It may have a significant personal and health service-related financial impact.

♦ It is mainly caused by cigarette smoking, but may occasionally occur in those who have never smoked.

What is COPD?

COPD is a long-term (chronic) disorder associated with reduced lung function, which does not change significantly over a short period of time. It is largely caused by cigarette smoking. The umbrella term 'COPD' now includes conditions previously known as:

♦ chronic obstructive airways disease;

♦ chronic airways disease;

♦   chronic bronchitis;

♦   emphysema.

These conditions can now be thought to be synonymous with COPD.

Individuals who develop COPD have abnormal and increased inflammation in the airways of the lung. This causes:

♦   an excess production of sticky mucus;

♦   destruction of areas of lung where oxygen passes into the bloodstream (making it more difficult to do so);

♦   difficulty in repairing damaged lung.

These changes all result in gradual narrowing of the airways, increased stiffness of the lungs (reduced compliance), and difficulty in exhaling all of the air within the lungs. This causes the lungs (and often the chest cavity) to increase in size over many years. As the disease progresses, the right side of the heart (which pumps blood into the lungs) can become overloaded and strained. This can cause fluid to collect around the ankles, but may later spread to involve the legs, lower back, abdomen, and liver. Doctors call this cor-pulmonale and it usually only occurs in advanced disease.

How common is COPD?

It is impossible to be certain precisely how many people in the UK, Europe, the USA, developing countries, and the world have COPD. What is known, is that the number of people currently diagnosed constitutes only the 'tip of the iceberg', as many others have not had a formal diagnosis. However, in the UK, COPD is thought to affect at least a million individuals.

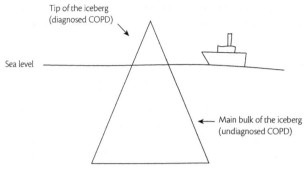

Fig. 2.1 Known cases of COPD may represent only the 'tip of the iceberg', with many individuals currently undiagnosed. In other words, these people live their life without knowing that they have the condition and often are unaware that any respiratory difficulty they may have is because of COPD.

Who does COPD affect?

The average age of diagnosis of COPD is in the late 60s and it becomes even more common with increasing age. COPD is more common in men, although the number of women being diagnosed is now increasing. It is also more common in socially deprived areas and in people living in developing countries. However, it can and does affect people of all walks of life, including the rich and famous!

How commonly do people die of COPD?

COPD is the fourth leading cause of death in the USA and Europe. With the increase in cigarette smoking in developing countries—especially China—it is expected that by 2020, it will become the third leading cause of death throughout the world. In the UK during 2003, there were approximately 26 000 deaths due to COPD—accounting for around 5% of all deaths. In the same year, 14 000 of these deaths were in men and 12 000 in women; in future years, it is thought that there will be no differences between men and women. On average in the UK, COPD reduces life expectancy by nearly 2 years; this number is even higher in those with more advanced disease. Between 10 and 20% of people with COPD are also thought to have coronary artery disease (narrowing of the arteries supplying the heart muscle).

What is the economic and heath resource impact of COPD?

Since the mid-1990s, emergency admissions to hospital for COPD have increased by at least 50%. Around 10% of all emergency admissions to hospital are due to worsening episodes of COPD, with this proportion even higher during winter months. Most of these admissions are in patients over 65 years of age with more advanced disease.

The vast majority of patients with COPD are looked after mainly by general practioners (GPs) and nurses in the community. On average, patients with COPD make six to seven visits annually to their GP. It has been estimated that each patient with diagnosed COPD costs the UK economy well over £1000 each year, which translates into over £900 million. The condition also results in personal financial losses due to the costs of disability in those with more advanced disease, absence from work, and premature retirement.

What are the causes of COPD?

Smoking

Cigarette smoking is the single most important risk factor in the development of COPD. Pipe and cigar smokers are also at an increased risk of developing it, although the risk is less than for cigarettes. Approximately 10–20% of individuals who smoke cigarettes develop significant COPD with symptoms. Although smoking is the most important risk factor, it can occur in non-smokers. For example, passive cigarette smoking (when an individual is exposed to cigarette smoke from a spouse, parent, work colleague, friend, or family member) can cause COPD. A condition very similar to COPD is also found in an uncommon disease called alpha-1 antitrypsin deficiency.

Air pollution

It is thought that air pollution may be involved to some extent in causing COPD. Studies have shown that higher levels of atmospheric air pollution are associated with cough, sputum production, breathlessness, and reduced lung function. In developing countries, indoor air pollution from fuel used for cooking and heating has been implicated as a risk factor for developing COPD, particularly in women.

Occupation

Some work environments with prolonged high exposure to some dusts and chemicals can cause COPD; examples include grain, coal, mineral dusts, and welding fumes. Cigarette smoking probably increases the risk of lung damage caused by some of these agents.

3

Making the diagnosis of COPD

Key points

- Typical symptoms of COPD include breathlessness, chest tightness, wheeze, cough, sputum production (especially in the mornings), reduced exercise capacity, and frequent chest infections.

- Many other medical conditions have features similar to COPD and need to be excluded.

- Breathing tests—known as spirometry—are required to diagnose COPD with certainty.

- A chest X-ray is needed at the time of diagnosis of COPD; this may be normal but helps to rule out other conditions.

Patients can be diagnosed with COPD by GPs, practice nurses, and hospital doctors. Who actually diagnoses it is unimportant; what is important is that a correct diagnosis is made and, once diagnosed, appropriate advice, education, non-drug and drug treatment, and follow-up appointments are provided.

History

Most consultations begin with speaking to patients to help find out what the problem might be. This is known as history taking and it is important that this is performed in a relaxed and unhurried manner. During this process, doctors and nurses ask many questions and they should allow ample time for responses to be considered and discussed. GPs or nurses may make an extra appointment to obtain all the relevant information, if insufficient time is initially available.

Features of COPD

COPD might be present in any patient over 35 years of age who has been, or still is, a cigarette smoker. Some individuals with very early or mild disease may have virtually no symptoms. However, as COPD progresses, you may develop any of the following symptoms (in isolation or in combination):

♦ breathlessness;

♦ chest tightness;

♦ wheeze;

♦ sputum production (especially in the mornings);

♦ cough;

♦ frequent winter chest infections;

♦ impaired exercise tolerance.

While these symptoms are consistent with COPD, they by no means confirm it. In order to be certain one way or another, definitive proof is necessary. This is achieved by asking the patient to perform specialized breathing tests known as spirometry with a machine called a spirometer (see below).

 Patient's perspective

Mr M, aged 52

I was struggling to shake off what I thought was a bad cough and went to the doctor to discover it was a chest infection. He then sent me to the practice nurse for some breathing tests. I was then referred to the hospital and diagnosed with COPD at the age of 42. Over time, I started to cough more than usual and started to get short of breath on exertion. My symptoms now are shortness of breath and tightening of the chest, feeling choked up, and tiredness

Conditions with features similar to COPD

Virtually any lung condition (e.g. asthma, bronchiectasis, lung fibrosis, and lung cancer) and many heart conditions (e.g. valve problems, heart muscle problems, and heart failure) can cause some of the symptoms of COPD. This all means that an accurate and careful history (what the patient tells the doctor or nurse) needs to be taken and definite proof that COPD is present (by way of breathing tests) is obtained. Asthma is often the main condition that doctors and nurses need to differentiate from COPD (especially in younger patients); features that may help distinguish between the two conditions are shown in Table 3.1.

Table 3.1 Differences between COPD and asthma

	COPD	Asthma
Age	>35 years	Any age
Cough	Persistent and productive	Intermittent and non-productive
Smoking	Almost invariable	Possible
Breathlessness	Progressive and persistent	Intermittent and variable
Night time symptoms	Uncommon unless in severe disease	Common
Family history	Uncommon unless family members also smoke	Common
Presence of eczema or hay fever	Possible	Common

 FAQ

Is it always possible to tell whether I have asthma or COPD?

No. Some patients with breathlessness and wheeze—who are or have been cigarette smokers—are discovered to have pure asthma and others pure COPD. In others, there may be some overlap between either condition. However, in patients who have some features of both asthma and COPD, the treatment is often similar.

 Patient perspective

Mr P, aged 74

In November 2006 I visited my GP as, once again, a cold had gone into my chest requiring a course of antibiotics. As a consequence of this visit,

I was subsequently diagnosed as having COPD. The diagnosis was made after having had some breathing tests (spirometry) and a chest X-ray. I immediately quit smoking.

I realize that smoking is the most likely cause of my COPD. Born into a post-Second World War era, the vast majority of adults at that time smoked cigarettes. By the age of 15 years, I had made the transition from 'sweetie cigarettes' to the tobacco variety. During the next 45 years I smoked between 20 and 30 cigarettes a day. I did make a number of attempts to quite over this time, but all of them ended in failure.

A year prior to the diagnosis of COPD, at the age of 58, I started to experience breathlessness both at home and at work when undertaking physical activities. Colds invariably went to my chest, requiring treatment with antibiotics, and while there was no change in my appetite, I lost a stone in weight.

Other aspects of assessment

As part of the overall assessment of COPD, doctors and nurses need to find out about:

- features of anxiety and depression;

- the presence of other medical conditions (such as heart disease, other chest problems, diabetes, high blood pressure);

- any allergies;

- current drugs and inhalers that the patient is taking (prescribed and not prescribed);

- frequency of exacerbations (episodes of worsening symptoms) of COPD;

- previous admissions to hospital;

- the distance that the patient can comfortably walk;

- what their occupation is (or was);

- present or past exposure to dusts or chemicals;

- number of days missed from work and associated financial losses;

- home circumstances;

- extent of social and family support;

- smoking status (and details about previous and current smoking habits);

- any previous vaccinations.

Smoking

Doctors and nurses also need to establish how many cigarettes have been smoked in a lifetime. This is often done by calculating the number of smoking-pack years. This can be done as follows:

Number of pack years
= (number of cigarettes smoked per day × number of years smoked) ÷ 20.

For example, a patient who has smoked 15 cigarettes per day for 40 years has a $(15 \times 40) \div 20 = 30$ pack year smoking history.

It is also useful to know if a spouse or any other family members currently smoke or have smoked cigarettes.

Examination

All patients with suspected COPD should be examined by a doctor. This should involve at least an examination of the lungs and also the heart. While the examination is often normal, features of other conditions that cause breathlessness—such as other lung or heart problems—may be discovered. Patient height and weight should also be recorded. This will enable the body mass index (BMI)—which is a measure of whether the patient's weight is within a healthy range or if they are under- or overweight—to be calculated. This is done by using the following equation:

Weight in kg divided by height squared in metres (height times your height).

For example, if a patient's weight is 70 kg and their height is 1.6 m:

BMI = $70 \div (1.6 \times 1.6) = 27$.

The BMI is classified for both males and females as follows:

♦ <18.5: underweight;

♦ 18.5–24.9: normal;

♦ 25–29.9: overweight;

♦ ≥30: obese.

Breathing tests

Breathing tests—known as spirometry—are essential in order to confirm or exclude the presence of COPD. These can be performed using a machine called a spirometer. They may be performed in many GP surgeries, specialized lung laboratories, hospital wards, or out-patient clinics.

The patient is asked to take a full breath inwards, and then blow out as hard and as fast as possible, for as long as possible, into a plastic tube attached to a recording device. This procedure is repeated several times until several recordings similar to one another have been measured. By evaluating these results and comparing them with values of a healthy individual, it can be determined whether the patient is likely to have COPD or not. Performing these breathing tests can also determine the severity of lung function impairment; this is usually divided into mild, moderate, or severe.

One of the most important parameters measured during spirometry is called the forced expiratory volume in 1 second and is abbreviated to FEV_1. This is the volume of air that can forcibly be breathed out in 1 second following a deep breath inwards. The expected FEV_1 in healthy people varies according to age, sex, and height; values obtained in patients with COPD are often compared with these 'predicted' values. This provides a percentage predicted value. Knowledge of the FEV_1—which is always impaired in COPD—helps to decide how severe COPD is and what treatment should be considered. In the UK, doctors and nurses classify the severity of COPD according to FEV_1 as follows:

♦ Significant COPD not present—FEV_1 80–100% of predicted (i.e. within normal limits).

♦ Mild disease—FEV_1 50–80% of predicted.

♦ Moderate disease—FEV_1 30–49% of predicted.

♦ Severe disease—FEV_1 <30% of predicted.

For example, if FEV$_1$ is measured at 2 litre and the expected value is 3 litre, then the FEV$_1$ will be 66% of predicted—this means that it falls into the mild category. Similarly, if FEV$_1$ is measured at 0.5 litre and the expected value is 2 litre, then the FEV$_1$ will be 25% of predicted—this means that it falls into the severe category.

You may be familiar with or have seen peak expiratory flow meters. These are useful in evaluating asthma, but are of less use in the diagnosis and monitoring of COPD.

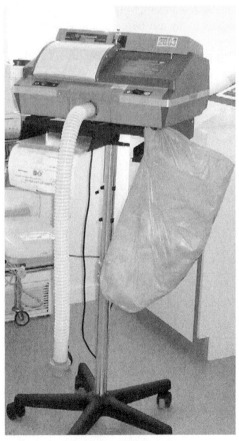

Fig. 3.1 A spirometer used to help diagnose COPD.

> **❓ FAQ**
>
> **Do I need to be seen in hospital before COPD can be diagnosed?**
>
> No. Many GP practices have spirometers that can be used to confirm the diagnosis in individuals with consistent symptoms.

Chest X-ray

All patients with suspected COPD should have a chest X-ray at the time of diagnosis. The chest X-ray can be normal in COPD, especially if there is mild disease. However, it is useful in identifying or suggesting other medical conditions that may cause some of the symptoms of COPD.

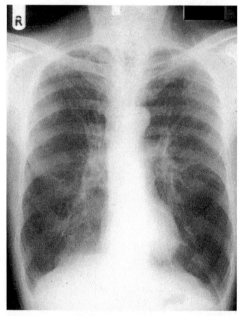

Fig. 3.2 A typical chest X-ray of a patient with COPD; this shows 'hyper-inflated' or 'enlarged' lung fields.

FAQ

What should happen if my chest X-ray is abnormal?

If your GP arranges a chest X-ray and it is abnormal, they may refer you to a chest specialist for further assessment and investigations.

Do I need repeat chest X-rays at regular intervals once COPD has been diagnosed?

No, this is not necessary. However, a chest X-ray may be repeated if you have particularly severe (or worrying) symptoms at any time.

Blood tests

There are no blood tests available to help diagnose COPD. However, since a low blood count (anaemia) can cause breathlessness on exertion and reduced ability to exercise, a blood test to exclude this should be performed at the time of investigation of symptoms or diagnosis.

When COPD is diagnosed in particularly young patients, or in those who have not smoked cigarettes to any great extent, doctors often need to exclude an uncommon condition that has similar features. This condition is called alpha-1 antitrypsin deficiency and can be easily excluded by a blood test. If it is discovered, checking to see if other family members have it and genetic counselling is necessary, as the condition can be inherited (passed on from generation to generation). It is imperative that individuals found to have alpha-1 antitrypsin deficiency do not smoke. Detailed information about this condition is outside the scope of this book but may be found on the following British Lung Foundation website: http://www.lunguk.org/you-and-your-lungs/conditions-and-diseases/alpha-1-antitrypsin.htm.

Other tests

Occasionally, other tests are required. For example, in advanced COPD, the heart can become strained and an electrocardiograph which is abbreviated to ECG (a heart tracing obtained by placing 12 leads on the chest and limbs) or echocardiogram (an ultrasound scan of the heart) may be performed. A minority of patients may have a more specialized investigation such as computed tomography (a CT scan) of their chest arranged if the diagnosis is uncertain, if the chest X-ray shows something of concern, or when a surgical procedure to the lungs is considered.

Some patients with COPD will have their oxygen levels checked from time to time using a hand-held device called a pulse oximeter (see Chapter 8). This is a simple test and involves placing a finger into a small plastic probe attached to a machine that gives an estimate of how much oxygen is being carried by the blood. The normal oxygen saturation is 97% and above; anything below this is abnormal. If levels are significantly low (e.g. less than 92%), an arterial blood gas may be required. This involves the doctor placing a small needle into an artery usually around the wrist. The exact level of oxygen and other dissolved gases can then be determined by placing the blood into a specialized machine called a blood gas analyser.

 FAQ

After being diagnosed with COPD, should I tell my partner?

Yes. It is often best to share worries, anxieties, and concerns with partners, family, and friends. Honesty and openness is usually the best policy! However, it is important that they do not take over your life and prevent you from doing what you enjoy doing, as exercising and keeping fit is one of the best treatments for COPD. On the other hand, do not be afraid to ask for help if you are finding difficulty in doing things you would like to do!

What measures can I take to avoid breathing in fumes and particles, which may worsen my breathing?

This is often difficult in real life, but it makes sense to stay away from people with colds and flu. You should also try to avoid parts of towns and cities where there is heavy traffic pollution and areas with lots of strong-smelling products and cigarette smoke. With legislation in the UK that bans smoking in public places, avoiding cigarette smoke when travelling on public transport and going out to restaurants, bars, shops, and the theatre has become far easier.

If I have COPD can I still have sex?

Yes. However, it should generally be avoided if you are particular breathless or immediately after a large meal, alcohol, or exercise.

Other than support provided by doctors and nurses is there any other help available?

Advice can be provided by the Breathe Easy network (email: breathe. easy@blf-uk.org). This network is a part of the British Lung Foundation and consists of small groups of individuals who provide support and information to anyone affected by lung problems such as COPD. These groups often meet on a regular basis and are an invaluable source of information and reassurance, and may arrange social events, talks, and exercise classes.

What should I do to see if I am entitled to support or benefits?

You should contact your local welfare support office for advice

4

Giving up smoking

> **➲ Key points**
>
> ♦ Cigarette smoking causes a range of chronic diseases and cancers.
>
> ♦ Smoking is by far the most important cause of COPD.
>
> ♦ Primary prevention of COPD involves preventing individuals from starting to smoke in the first place.
>
> ♦ Smoking cessation is vital in the successful management of COPD.
>
> ♦ Willpower and determination are required to stop smoking; you usually need to feel that the time is right for you to stop.
>
> ♦ Smoking cessation aids include counselling, nicotine replacement therapy, and some specific drugs (the most common ones being Zyban/bupropion and Champix/varenicline).

Smoking was first introduced into the UK in the sixteenth century, and its popularity has continued to increase. Apart from being the most important cause of COPD, cigarette smoking can also cause or contribute towards a range of other chronic (long-term) diseases and cancers affecting almost every part of the body. Examples of these include:

Cancers:

♦ lung;

♦ throat;

- gullet;

- bladder;

- kidney;

- stomach;

- pancreatic.

Chronic diseases and conditions:

- heart disease (angina and heart failure);

- high blood pressure;

- strokes and mini strokes;

- narrowing of the leg arteries (peripheral vascular disease);

- breakdown of the retina in the eye (macular degeneration);

- osteoporosis.

Smoking is also associated with:

- persistent symptoms of asthma;

- lung infections and pneumonia;

- greater chance of developing complications with diabetes;

- infertility and impotence;

- premature ageing;

- increased skin wrinkling.

Cigarette smoking delivers high doses of nicotine, which is a powerfully addictive drug, quickly and directly to the brain. Addiction to nicotine is usually established following experimentation with cigarettes during adolescence and may result in lifelong smoking. Nicotine itself does not cause major health problems in most users; it is the tar that accompanies nicotine that accounts for most of the harm caused by cigarettes.

Patient's perspective

Mr P, aged 74

I was 8 years old when I started smoking. I got two old pennies for my pocket money on a Saturday to go to the pictures. Instead, I went to one of the local shops, which had a cigarette machine outside. I put one old penny in the machine and received two cigarettes, two matches, and even some change! This went on for 3–4 years until the war broke out and the machine was removed—this was my introduction to smoking. With hindsight, this was all a bit of 'bravado' and me pretending to be a grown up. As the years went by, I began to smoke more and more, and was soon up to smoking 20 cigarettes a day. I did give up for a couple of years when I was 16 years old. This was because I was admitted to hospital for a prolonged period of time and cigarettes were not allowed. At 18 years old, I started smoking in earnest. I actually quite enjoyed doing it as it helped if there was any stress at work.

I began to feel breathless and have a tight chest during exertion; I also noticed a worsening cough and I produced a lot of sputum. At this point, I was referred to a clinic at my local hospital and was given an appointment with a consultant chest specialist. He diagnosed COPD after speaking to me, examining me, and asking me to breathe into a tube attached to a machine, which gave a printout. I was advised to immediately stop smoking. I did manage to successfully do this with the help of nicotine replacement patches. I stopped smoking in 2000; this was around 65 years after starting.

I was retired when COPD was diagnosed. This was quite convenient as I was walking much slower. I also needed more time to walk the dog in the mornings, and wash and dress myself. I came to realize in the years after being diagnosed with COPD that I wasn't going to get an awful lot better.

Preventing people from smoking

Primary prevention involves adopting different measures to try and prevent people from starting to smoke in the first place. This usually prevents the development of COPD. The most effective approach to primary prevention is the widespread use of strategies that reduce incentives to smoke. Examples of these include:

♦ bans on cigarette advertising and promotion;

♦ increases in the price of cigarettes;

♦ policing of illegal sources of cheap cigarettes;

♦ smoke-free policies at work and in public places;

♦ health warnings on cigarette packs;

♦ health promotion campaigns.

Smoking cessation

Smoking cessation should underpin the management of all patients with COPD who continue to smoke. This is important irrespective of age, the length of time that someone has smoked, the quantity of cigarettes smoked, and the severity of symptoms. Individuals who quit smoking benefit from a significant improvement in overall health, social and emotional well-being, and survival. It also reduces the chance of developing other chronic diseases and cancers in the future. In addition to sheer determination and willpower, smokers can be helped to stop smoking by a combination of counselling, nicotine replacement therapy, and some specific drugs.

It is fairly well established that everyone (healthy and otherwise) over the age of 30 has a slow and age-related decline in lung function. Large scientific

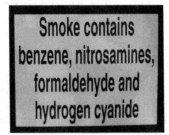

Fig. 4.1 Warnings found on cigarette packets are useful ways in which to remind individuals of the dangers of smoking.

studies have shown that continued cigarette smoking accelerates this rate of decline in lung function. Reassuringly, the rate of decline changes back to that of a non-smoker after cessation, irrespective of the age of quitting. It is therefore important to emphasize to all patients with COPD (and even those without the condition) that it is never too late to stop smoking.

 FAQ

What is nicotine?

Tobacco comes from a plant called *Nicotiana tabacum*. For many hundreds of years, people have smoked and chewed tobacco leaves from this plant.

Why do people smoke?

Nicotine affects areas of the brain that produce feelings of pleasure and contentedness. In particular, it can raise the level of a substance in the brain called dopamine, which helps create a general air of well-being.

Why is it difficult to stop smoking?

Nicotine is addictive. This means that when it is removed from the body, people usually experience withdrawal symptoms such as restlessness, unhappiness, hunger, headaches, difficulty sleeping, irritability, and they can become generally ill at ease.

Counselling

Doctors and nurses should encourage the patient (and everyone else who smokes) to quit at every available opportunity; advice should be offered in an encouraging, non-judgemental, and friendly manner. Smoking cessation is not easy and several attempts may be required before long-term success is achieved. The following tips may be of some use in helping to achieve success:

♦ aim to stop smoking completely;

♦ set a date;

♦ ask family and friends to support a quit attempt;

◆ consider what has and hasn't helped in previous attempts to quit;

◆ get rid of all cigarettes;

◆ develop the idea that cigarettes kill;

◆ appreciate the fact that cigarette smoking confers pleasure mainly because it prevents withdrawal symptoms;

◆ list harmful chemicals that are found in cigarettes;

◆ list diseases that cigarette smoking cause;

◆ be aware that most withdrawal symptoms pass within about a month;

◆ create goals and rewards for success;

◆ devise coping mechanisms to use during periods of craving;

◆ encourage partners, friends, and work colleagues to quit at the same time;

◆ use nicotine replacement therapy;

◆ make use of follow-up support by nurses, counsellors, and doctors.

Nicotine replacement therapy

Nicotine replacement therapy is the most commonly used aid to help individuals to stop smoking. It works by replacing the supply of nicotine, without delivery of the harmful components of cigarette smoke.

Although some forms of nicotine replacement therapy (gum, inhalator, nose spray, or lozenges) deliver nicotine more quickly than others (skin patches), all deliver a lower total dose, and deliver it to the brain more slowly than a cigarette. Since none of these methods of delivering nicotine is generally better (or worse) than the other, the best approach is to choose which product you prefer. However, if you are a heavy cigarette smoker, a slow-release product (such as a skin patch) plus a fast-acting product for periods of craving may be of greater benefit. If you are a light smoker (less than 10 cigarettes per day), or if you wait longer than an hour before your first cigarette of the day, it might be preferable to use a short-acting product in advance of your regular cigarettes or at times of craving.

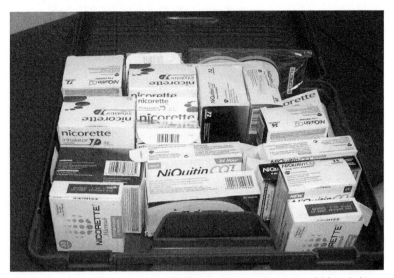

Fig. 4.2 A variety of nicotine replacement therapy preparations are available to help patients quit smoking.

Treatment with nicotine replacement therapy is generally recommended for up to 3 months. This should be followed by a gradual withdrawal. Nicotine replacement therapy is generally well tolerated, although side-effects include:

◆ nausea;

◆ headache;

◆ unpleasant taste;

◆ hiccoughs;

◆ indigestion;

◆ sore throat;

◆ palpitations (an awareness of your heart beat);

◆ dizziness;

◆ difficulty sleeping;

◆ nasal irritation and bleeding (if using the spray).

It should also be used with caution if you have any of the following conditions:

◆ overactive thyroid gland;

◆ diabetes;

◆ kidney problems;

◆ liver problems;

◆ stomach ulceration;

◆ narrowing of the arteries of the legs (peripheral vascular disease);

◆ skin disorders (avoid patches);

◆ severe heart problems and after a heart attack;

◆ recent stroke;

◆ pregnancy and breastfeeding.

Drugs

Bupropion (Zyban)

Bupropion is an antidepressant, although it is effective even if you are not depressed. It is generally as useful as nicotine replacement therapy in terms of smoking cessation rates. There is nothing to suggest that using nicotine replacement therapy and bupropion at the same time is of any benefit. Bupropion helps to prevent weight gain, which is commonly associated with quitting. The main adverse effect is its association with fits (convulsions) and it should not be used if you have a past history of epilepsy and seizures. It should also be used with caution, or even avoided, in the following situations:

◆ use of drugs that interact with it (such as some antidepressants, malaria tablets, antihistamines, and theophylline);

◆ alcohol or benzodiazepine drug withdrawal;

◆ eating disorders;

- bipolar illness;

- brain tumours;

- pregnancy and breastfeeding;

- severe liver disease.

Unlike nicotine replacement therapy (which is usually started at the same time as a quit attempt) bupropion should start 1 or 2 weeks earlier. It should be stopped if cessation has not been achieved within 8 weeks.

Varenicline (Champix)

Varenicline is a relatively new drug available for help in smoking cessation. It should only be used if you have expressed a real wish to stop smoking. Like bupropion, it should be started 1–2 weeks before the quit date and the dose slowly increased over a 3-month period. It should be avoided in pregnancy and breastfeeding women, and used with caution in kidney disease (although it may be used in a lower dose) and those with a history of psychiatric disorders. Side-effects include:

- bowel upset and altered appetite;

- dry mouth and taste disturbance;

- headache;

- drowsiness;

- dizziness;

- sleep disorders;

- abnormal dreams.

Patient's perspective

Mr M, aged 52

I was 14 when I started smoking, for no other reason than all my friends were. I started on 2 cigarettes a day, then 5; by the time I left school at 15 and had a job and was receiving a wage, I was smoking 20 a day. I progressed from there to 40 cigarettes each day. I stopped smoking only after being diagnosed with COPD at the hospital. On my second appointment, the doctor looked at me and asked if I had stopped smoking yet. I got the impression he was saying you are here for me to help you, but you have to help yourself first. I totally agreed. I vowed to myself that on my next appointment I would be able to tell him that I had stopped. I did manage to stop smoking and that was me, a non-smoker forever. If I did not stop smoking when I did, I have no doubt at all that things would be looking very bleak and feel it is something you must do as soon as possible.

 FAQ

How long do the effects of smoking a cigarette last?

After inhaling a cigarette, nicotine is absorbed by the lungs, passes into the bloodstream and reaches the brain in less than 10 seconds. The effects of nicotine from a cigarette can last several hours. It can easily be seen that smoking a single cigarette may therefore lead to people smoking more and more each day in order to achieve more longer lasting effects.

Where do I get help to stop smoking?

In addition to speaking to your doctor or nurse, you may wish to contact the smoking advice service (SAS). The SAS provides free advice and support to anyone looking for help in quitting. It consists of smoking-cessation advisors who are trained in helping you with all aspects of giving up; they can be contacted on freephone 0500 600 332.

5

Managing COPD without drugs

⮕ Key points

♦ Non-drug treatment plays a vital role in the management of COPD.

♦ A variety of health care professionals may offer different forms of help in the management of COPD.

♦ Examples of non-drug treatment include education, pulmonary rehabilitation, vaccination, encouragement of exercise, and dietary advice.

♦ Anxiety and depression are common in COPD; all doctors and nurses should look for them and treat accordingly.

♦ Surgical procedures have a limited role in the routine management of COPD.

The ultimate aims of COPD management are varied and incorporate a variety of ideals. Some of these include:

♦ a reduction in symptoms;

♦ an improvement in exercise tolerance;

♦ an improvement in quality of life;

♦ prevention of exacerbations;

♦ a level of care and treatment that patients find satisfactory for their individual needs;

◆ provision of a drug regime that maximizes gain and minimizes the risk of side-effects;

◆ living longer with the disease and maintaining a good quality of life;

◆ slowing the progression of disease.

Non-drug treatment (everything else other than inhalers or tablets) plays a vital role in the overall management of COPD. This aspect of management is often underestimated and underused by patients, nurses, and doctors, and underresourced. It could be argued that non-drug treatment is at least as important as drug treatment.

Who will be involved in my care?

Many different types of health care professionals are important in delivering care to patients with COPD. These individuals are referred to as the multidisciplinary team and they can greatly assist patients with different physical, domestic, and social limitations caused by COPD. Respiratory nurse specialists are likely to have an increasingly important role in patient management and can provide a vital link between primary care (everything provided by GPs) and secondary care (everything provided by hospitals). The role of respiratory nurse specialists is likely to vary considerably between health care regions, but potentially important areas where they can provide support include:

◆ helping to deal with emotional and psychological aspects of the disease;

◆ better understanding and knowledge of COPD and its treatment;

◆ assessing and correcting inhaler technique;

◆ nebulizer assessments;

◆ organization of early discharge or assisted discharge schemes (see Chapter 9);

◆ end of life symptom management;

◆ family support.

Other members of the multidisciplinary team are decribed below.

Physiotherapists

They may help patients get 'back on their feet' following an exacerbation, provide advice on breathing exercises and relaxation techniques, and run pulmonary rehabilitation programmes.

Dieticians

They may advise patients regarding the best diet for their individual needs. This involves education about the best diet for a particular patient, practical help regarding appropriate foodstuffs, and provision of high-energy drinks supplements, where necessary.

Occupational therapists

They may assess home surroundings and the ability of patients to look after themselves. If necessary, they may help to adapt homes, and to provide practical tools and aids to enable patients to cope more easily.

Social workers

They may help to find practical solutions regarding changes in home circumstances. For example, social workers can offer assistance in moving to a more suitable house, organize care services for a relative, and provide advice regarding financial and social matters.

Pharmacists

They are involved in dispensing tablets and inhalers and can advise on how to use inhalers correctly. They also offer advice on potential drug interactions, side-effects of drugs, ways to stop smoking, and help keep track of drug prescriptions and potential changes.

Mental health care workers

They may help discuss psychological aspects of COPD and how it affects the patient. They may advise on relaxation techniques and coping strategies, and offer counselling sessions.

Doctors

They manage overall care and help to co-ordinate treatment and management decisions

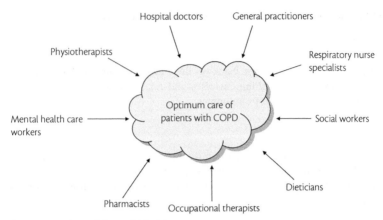

Fig. 5.1 Members of the multidisciplinary team.

Pulmonary rehabilitation

Most patients—irrespective of age, severity of symptoms, and whether they smoke—should be referred to a pulmonary rehabilitation class, if at all possible. Pulmonary rehabilitation is a specially organized programme for patients with chronic respiratory disorders, which is designed to improve physical, psychological, and social well-being. These programmes, with an emphasis on graded or gradual exercise, may help to break the vicious circle of breathlessness, inactivity, and reduced fitness, which is only too often encountered. Pulmonary rehabilitation may be especially useful following an acute exacerbation of COPD in terms of improving exercise capacity and overall general health. The ideal programme should consist of several components, including exercise training, education, and nutritional advice.

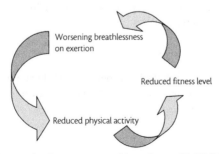

Fig. 5.2 The vicious cycle often encountered in patients with COPD.

Exercise training

Regular moderate exercise is of benefit to both healthy people and those with most chronic diseases. In COPD, regular physical activity is associated with a variety of physical and psychological advantages. Many hospitals run out-patient rehabilitation programmes, and if you are offered a place on one, it is advisable to attend if at all possible. Exercise training as part of a pulmonary rehabilitation programme can:

♦ improve the distance a patient can walk;

♦ improve muscle strength;

♦ improve quality of life;

♦ reduce symptoms.

Typical out-patient pulmonary rehabilitation programmes run for around 2 months, with supervised exercise classes taking place 2–3 times a week. They are usually, but not always, run by a dedicated team of physiotherapists. Patients are also encouraged to exercise at home and to complete records, so that progress can be monitored and discussed. On the whole, any benefit gained will match the amount of effort put in.

Education

Pulmonary rehabilitation also provides the opportunity for further education about the condition. In addition to helping develop a greater understanding of what is actually wrong, education should also consist of:

♦ breathing control exercises;

♦ relaxation techniques;

♦ an emphasis on the benefits of exercise and the value of smoking cessation.

Patients should be made aware of different breathing techniques, which may help them to cope with breathlessness. For example, it is important to learn to control breathing patterns by means of using the least effort possible with relaxed shoulders, arms, and hands. One technique is relaxed and slow, deep breathing. This involves slowing down the breathing rate and taking deep breathes in through the nose and out through the mouth. It may also be help-ful to purse the lips when breathing out (lips should be positioned as if whis-tling). Another technique involves co-ordinating breaths in time with steps.

For example, when going up stairs, it might be helpful to breathe in for 2 steps and out for 3 steps. There are also some positions that may be useful to adopt when particularly short of breath (Figure 5.3).

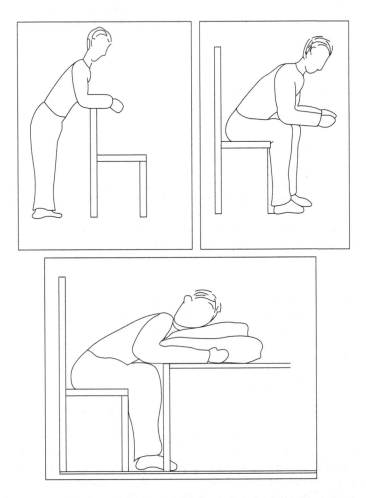

Fig. 5.3 A variety of different positions—which use little energy and require little effort—can be adopted when you are particularly breathless. Try all of these and consider which one is best; depending on circumstances, one may be preferable over another.

Nutritional advice

Many patients with COPD are underweight. This in part may be due to increased calorie requirements due to the work of breathing. Social isolation and reduced nutritional intake due to limitations caused by severe breathlessness may also mean that some patients fail to eat regular meals. In contrast, patients may become overweight due to reduced physical activity and overeating, often due to boredom.

All patients with COPD should have their BMI calculated (see Chapter 3). Advice on an appropriate diet should then be arranged, if patients are found to be underweight (BMI <18.5) or obese (BMI >30). As well as general advice as to what sorts of food patients should eat, supplemental drinks, high in calories, can be given where necessary.

In terms of diet, general principles include:

◆ eating a variety of foods;

◆ balancing the amount of food eaten against the amount of physical activity;

◆ eating plenty of fresh fruit and vegetables;

◆ choosing a diet low in fat, especially saturated fat and cholesterol; to help do this, grill instead of frying foods, use low fat margarine and milk, and trim fat from any meat eaten;

◆ reducing sugar intake;

◆ taking plenty of vitamins.

Vaccination

Many exacerbations of COPD are caused by viruses and bacteria. This means that specific vaccines may play an important role in the prevention of exacerbations. Two main vaccines have been developed and are active against a common strain of bacteria that can produce pneumonia (pneumococcal vaccination) and the flu (influenza vaccination).

Pneumococcal vaccination

A particular bacterium called *Streptococcus pneumoniae* is one of the most common causes of pneumonia in the UK. In view of this, a vaccine has been developed against this particular bacterium and should be offered to most patients with COPD. A single dose is given by injection into an arm or leg muscle;

revaccination is generally not recommended. Mild soreness and swelling at the site of injection is a common occurrence.

Influenza vaccination

All patients with COPD should be offered annual influenza vaccination. Since it is prepared from parts of chick embryos, it should not be given if you have an egg allergy. Influenza vaccine is prepared each year using viruses similar to those considered most likely to be circulating in the forthcoming winter. Patients are often concerned about side-effects and may have doubts about the benefits of the vaccine. However, it is considered to be effective in reducing exacerbation rates of COPD and prevention of pneumonia and hospital admissions. The vaccine is usually given by an injection into an upper arm or leg muscle.

Table 5.1 Hospital Anxiety and Depression scale

Anxiety	
I feel tense or wound up:	Most of the time–3, a lot of the time–2, from time to time–1, not at all–0.
I get sort of frightened feelings as if something awful is going to happen:	Definitely and badly–3, yes but not too badly–2, a little–1, not at all–0
Worrying thoughts go through my mind:	Very definitely–3, yes but not too badly–2, a little–1, not at all–0
I can sit at ease and feel relaxed:	Definitely–0, usually–1, not often–2, not at all–3
I get a sort of frightened feeling like butterflies in the stomach:	Not at all–0, occasionnally–1, quite often–2, very often–3
I feel restless as if I have to be on the move:	Very much indeed–3, quite a lot–2, not very much–1, not at all–0
I get sudden feelings of panic:	Very often indeed–3, quite often–2, not very often–1, not at all–0
Depression	
I look forward with enjoyment to things:	As much as I ever did–0, rather less than I used to–1, definitely less than I used to–2, hardly at all–3
I have lost interest in my appearance:	Definitely–3, I take not so much care as I should–2, I may not take quite as much care–1, I take as much care as ever–0
I still enjoy the things I used to enjoy:	Definitely as much–0, not quite so much–1, only a little–2, hardly at all–3

Table 5.1 Hospital Anxiety and Depression scale *(continued)*

Depression	
I can laugh and see the funny side of things:	As much as I always could–0, not quite so much–1, definitely not so much–2, not at all–3
I feel cheerful:	Not at all–3, not often–2, sometimes–1, most of the time–0
I feel as if I am slowed down:	Nearly all the time–3, very often–2, sometimes–1, not at all–0
I can enjoy a good book, the radio, or a TV programme:	Often–0, sometimes–1, not often–2, seldom–3

Scoring is based on a 4-point scale (0–3). An overall score in either category of 0–7 is normal, 8–10 borderline, and 11–21 suggests moderate to severe anxiety or depression.

Anxiety and depression

Anxiety and depression are often found in patients with COPD. If present, these may further impair physical, emotional, and social well-being. These conditions are probably caused by a variety of factors such as isolation, persistent breathlessness, and increasing difficulty in participation in daily activities such as meeting friends and family, shopping, travelling, and exercising. In view of this, doctors and nurses should try and identify features suggestive of an anxiety or depressive disorder. Mental health status can be assessed with a simple questionnaire such as the Hospital Anxiety and Depression scale (Table 5.1). If patients are found to have anxiety or depression, it should be treated the same way as in patients who don't have COPD. This should usually be with a combination of relaxation techniques, talking therapies (counselling and cognitive behavioural therapy), and medications such as antidepressants and drugs to relieve anxiety.

Surgery

Surgical procedures to the lung in an attempt to reduce symptoms in COPD are not often performed. However, there are some circumstances when a surgeon could be asked to consider one of several procedures. These are not without risk, and patients should keep in mind the fact that there is always a risk of serious complications during any surgical procedure or general anaesthetic. The actual risks vary widely from person to person and beween different operations. These should generally be discussed in full with the surgeon along with family and friends.

Lung volume reduction surgery

Lung volume reduction surgery (LVRS) involves removing inefficient parts of the lung, leaving more efficient parts to work more effectively. Studies have shown that this form of surgery can improve quality of life, exercise capacity, and lung function in carefully selected people. It is a safer procedure than lung transplantation and avoids the problem of lack of donor lungs. LVRS should be considered in patients with very poor lung function, COPD mainly affecting the upper parts of the lung, and poor exercise tolerance. A further procedure with principles similar to LVRS has been developed but does not involve surgery (bronchoscopic lung volume reduction). This involves placing one-way valves into the lung, which causes the most inefficient parts of the lung to reduce in size, leaving the more efficient parts plenty of room to perform the work of breathing. However, further studies to investigate more fully this technique are required.

Bullectomy

In some patients with COPD, a large non-functioning air sac (called a bulla) can occupy a relatively large volume of lung. This can cause compression of surrounding efficiently working lung. In patients with a large air sac, especially those with persistent symptoms, a previously collapsed lung (pneumothorax), or who have coughed up blood, an operation to remove the air sac (bullectomy) can be considered.

Transplantation

Some motivated individuals with advanced COPD can be considered for lung transplantation. However, as with most transplant procedures, this is greatly limited by the number of donor lungs available. Older patients with other medical conditions (such as heart disease, diabetes, and kidney disorders) generally have poorer survival rates. It is generally considered that the upper age limit for a double lung transplant (both lungs) is 60 years and for a single lung transplant (only one lung) is 65 years. Lung transplantation may be considered in patients with:

♦ very advanced disease;

♦ severe difficulty in coping with everyday living activities;

♦ an anticipated life expectancy of <2 years.

Lung transplantation is not without short- and long-term potential problems. For example, there is a risk of dying either during or immediately after the procedure, and patients need to be maintained on powerful antirejection drugs (which can cause problems of their own) for the rest of their life. There are only a handful of hospitals in the UK that perform lung transplant procedures. Before being considered for a lung transplant, individuals need to be thoroughly assessed over several days; this usually takes place at the transplant centre.

6

Managing COPD with drugs

⮕ Key points

♦ All patients with COPD should have a reliever inhaler for use on an 'as required' basis; these drugs open up the airway and are called short-acting bronchodilators.

♦ Individuals with persistent symptoms should use a preventer inhaler on a daily basis; these drugs also open up the airway and are called long-acting bronchodilators.

♦ A further type of inhaled drug called inhaled steroids should be considered in cases of frequent exacerbations and more advanced disease.

♦ Theophylline tablets now play a limited role in COPD and are often associated with troublesome side-effects.

♦ Steroid tablets should not be used on a long-term basis if at all possible, since they are associated with multiple side-effects. However, they may be considered in a minority of patients.

Drug treatment plays an important role in the management of COPD. However, it cannot be emphasized enough that non-drug treatment (as highlighted in the previous chapter) should also take place at the same time. The different drugs used in COPD should usually be started in a gradual and stepwise manner, with a follow-up review appointment made to discuss the patient's thoughts and opinions and any benefit or side-effects. The decision to use different types of inhaled and oral drugs is usually made on the basis of patient preference, the degree of lung function impairment, severity and persistence of symptoms, how far and how long the patient can exercise, and the frequency of exacerbations. In other words, those with more mild disease need fewer inhaled drugs, while those with more advanced disease need more drugs.

The most effective drug treatment in COPD tends to be delivered by inhaler devices. Inhaled drugs are usually divided into:

◆ 'relievers', which should be taken on an *intermittent* basis to provide rapid *relief* of symptoms (often within minutes); and

◆ 'preventers', which should be used on a *daily* basis to *prevent* symptoms and exacerbations.

Inhaled short-acting bronchodilators

COPD sufferers should carry a reliever inhaler at all times. This type of inhaler should usually be used 'if and when' there are more symptoms than normal. The type of drug used to relieve symptoms rapidly is called a short-acting bronchodilator. These types of drugs rapidly (usually within minutes) open the airways within the chest and reduce symptoms such as breathlessness, wheeze, and chest tightness. The two main types of short-acting bronchodilator drugs are called short-acting β_2-agonists and short-acting anticholinergics, and may be used alone or together in the same inhaler device. Both of these types of drug have effects lasting up to 4–6 h. They are both are well tolerated, but may cause tremor of the hands or palpitations (an increased awareness of your heart beat).

Inhaled long-acting bronchodilators

In patients with more persistent symptoms and exacerbations, a longer acting drug to try and prevent these problems should be given. These types of drugs are called long-acting bronchodilators of which there are two main types: a long-acting β_2-agonist or long-acting anticholinergic. Both of these types of drug are effective in opening the airways for 12–24 h and can be used alone or in combination.

Long-acting β_2-agonists

The two most commonly used types of long-acting β_2-agonist are called salmeterol and formoterol; their effects last up to 12 h. They are both widely used and very safe, although some of their side-effects include:

◆ fast heart beat and palpitations;

◆ tremor;

◆ headache;

◆ muscle cramps;

◆ low potassium in the bloodstream;

◆ feeling of nervousness and jitteriness.

Long-acting anticholinergic

The only inhaled long-acting anticholinergic drug used is called tiotropium (Spiriva). It should be taken once a day and its effects last for up to 24 h. Some of its side-effects include:

◆ dry mouth;

◆ nausea;

◆ constipation;

◆ headache;

◆ fast heart beat and palpitations;

◆ visual difficulties;

◆ difficulty in passing urine.

 FAQ

Are inhalers containing steroids safe?

Inhaled steroids are generally safe in the doses used in COPD. In higher doses, the most common problems include an alteration in the quality of your voice, and thrush (a fungal infection characterized by white patches within the mouth and around the gums).

Do inhalers containing steroids cause weight gain?

As a general rule no.

Do the constituents of inhalers damage the ozone layer?

The vast majority of inhalers used nowadays have no harmful effect upon the ozone layer. Previously, the propellants used to help deliver drugs to the lungs (called chlorofluorocarbons) were thought to cause some damage to the ozone layer, but these have now been phased out in the UK.

How do I know if my inhaler has run out?

Some inhalers (e.g. Turbohalers and Accuhalers) contain a counter that tells you how many doses are left. In those that do not have a counter, you will know it is empty as no sound is made when it is shaken.

What happens if I miss a dose of inhaled drug?

This doesn't really matter, just continue to take your next dose as normal. If, however, you do remember within a few hours, there is no harm in taking your missed dose at that point.

Inhaled steroids

Inhaled steroids play a major role in the treatment of asthma, but are far less beneficial in COPD. They should be considered in those with more advanced disease and repeated exacerbations. They do not have any great impact upon improving lung function or symptoms, but may reduce the frequency of exacerbations. Commonly used inhaled steroids are called beclomethasone, budesonide, and fluticasone.

Inhaled steroids can cause side-effects to appear within the mouth and throat, and in other parts of the body. Within the mouth and throat they may cause thrush; this appears as white plaques on the tongue and insides of the mouth, and is caused by a fungal infection. It can be easily treated with antifungal mouth drops, lozenges, or tablets. Inhaled steroids may also cause an alteration in voice quality; this can be prevented or treated by gargling and brushing your teeth after using inhaled steroids, using a spacer device (see below), and using a smaller dose of drug. Studies have also suggested that prolonged use of high doses of inhaled steroids may cause the skin to bruise more easily and osteoporosis (thinning of the bones). Inhaled steroids should usually not be stopped suddenly as doing so can cause the adrenal gland (located within the abdomen on top of the kidneys) to stop making its own form of steroid, which can cause serious problems.

Combined inhaled steroid and long-acting β_2-agonist inhalers

Inhaled steroids should not generally be used alone in COPD; they are most often given along with a long-acting β_2-agonist in a single inhaler. This in turn may increase the likelihood of using the inhaler every day, as one inhaler is easier and quicker to use than two.

Table 6.1 The main combination inhalers containing two different types of drug used in COPD

Name of combination inhaler	Steroid and long-acting β_2-agonist
Symbicort	Budesonide + Formoterol
Seretide	Fluticasone + Salmeterol

Theophylline

Theophylline is one of the oldest treatments still used for COPD. It works by opening the airways and is usually given twice a day. Inhaled drugs form the mainstay of treatment, but in patients with more advanced disease and persistent symptoms, theophylline should be added on a trial basis. It is usually started in a low dose and, if tolerated, the dose should be increased a week or so later.

Side-effects are fairly common with theophylline. Examples of some of these include:

◆ fast and irregular heart beat;

◆ nausea and vomiting;

◆ abdominal pain;

◆ diarrhoea;

◆ headache;

◆ seizures;

◆ low potassium in the bloodstream.

Some drugs (such as some anticonvulsants, antidepressants, antibiotics, lithium, verapamil, diltiazem, St John's Wort, and fluconazole) and medical conditions (such as heart failure, liver cirrhosis, and current cigarette smoking) can alter how the body breaks down (metabolizes) theophylline. This means that theophylline levels may rise (and cause side-effects to appear) or fall (causing it to be less effective). Doctors, pharmacists, and nurses therefore need to remain vigilant when patients are using theophylline blood levels 4–6 h after taking a dose may need to be checked on occasion.

Steroids tablets

Daily steroid tablets have a very limited role in the management of COPD (other than during an exacerbation). As a general rule, using steroids tablets on a long-term basis should be avoided. However, some patients find it difficult to discontinue steroids completely following an exacerbation. This is usually due to a recurrence of the symptoms that required them to be prescribed in the first place. In situations where withdrawal of steroid tablets is impossible, the lowest possible dose (e.g. 5 mg of prednisolone/day) may be used on a long-term basis.

Before starting long-term steroids, patients should be aware that they must not be stopped suddenly and that a slow reduction in dose is usually necessary. If steroids are withdrawn suddenly after prolonged periods of use, the adrenal glands may suddenly stop making their own natural steroid hormone,

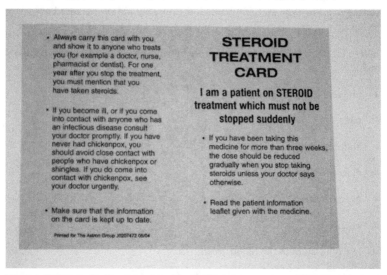

Fig. 6.1 Patients using long-term steroids should carry a warning card letting others know what treatment they are receiving.

which can lead to serious problems (called adrenal insufficiency). In view of this, all patients receiving oral steroids should be given a treatment card alerting others of the problems associated with abruptly stopping them. Courses of oral steroids that last less than 3 weeks (e.g. given to treat an exacerbation of COPD) do not generally require to be gradually reduced before stopping.

When used for a prolonged period of time, steroids can be associated with a variety of side-effects, such as osteoporosis. To counteract this particular problem, tablets to prevent it can be given. These are called bisphosphonates and should be used with calcium supplements.

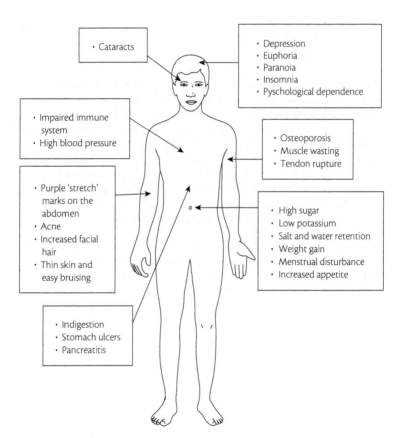

Fig. 6.2 Long-term use of steroid tablets can be associated with a variety of side-effects.

Patient's perspective

Mr M, aged 52

My treatment currently consists of combivent nebulules, ventolin evohaler, Seretide, Spiriva, and uniphyllin tablets. I don't have any problems taking my medicine. On average I have treatment with antibiotics and steroids about four times a year. I attend the hospital twice a year as an out-patient. As yet I have never been admitted to hospital.

 Patient's perspective

Mr P, aged 74

At the moment my treatment consists of Seretide 500, one puff twice a day, and Spiriva, one suck a day; I use Ventolin if and when I need to take it. I have had no problems or side-effects with my inhaled treatment. I often need courses of antibiotics and steroids for exacerbations of COPD and have had around six lots in the past year. I have recently had a scare as I was found to have a 'shadow' on my lung and needed a bronchoscopy (a flexible telescope passed down into my lungs) and CT scan of my chest. Luckily, I did not have cancer, but the changes noted on my chest X-ray were probably due to the fact that I had been exposed to asbestos early on in my working career in the shipyards.

This year has not been so good for me as I needed to be admitted to hospital on two separate occasions for pneumonia. It has taken me a while to recover from these episodes and I often worry as to whether I will have a recurrence in the future.

Patient's perspective

Mt Q, aged 62

Medication (Seretide) for the condition was prescribed a year later as I continued to suffer breathlessness from physical activities such as walking up an incline, climbing stairs, dressing, i.e. most activities requiring physical effort. As I was concerned at the worsening of the condition and the possible outcomes, I was referred to a chest specialist.

The outcome from the referral was that my COPD was considered to be mild in severity, based on my lung function tests. I was also reassured that as long as I refrained from smoking, the condition should not get worse and the prognosis in general was good. It was also suggested that I change to Spiriva every day (instead of Seretide) together with Ventolin as required, as my COPD is only mild.

Other drugs

Mucolytics

Sputum overproduction is commonly found in patients with COPD. A class of drug called mucolytics is thought to reduce the viscosity (thickness) of sputum in the airways and helps in coughing it out. Although it is unclear as to whether this class of drugs provides any great benefit, they may be tried if the patient has a cough producing lots of thick, sticky sputum and is troubled by frequent exacerbations. Examples of this type of drug include carbocysteine, erdocysteine, and mecysteine. These drugs are well tolerated and have few side-effects.

Diuretics

Diuretics (commonly referred to as 'water tablets') are designed to remove excess fluid from the body. In some patients with COPD—usually with more advanced disease—fluid retention around the lower legs can be a problem. In such circumstances, a small dose of diuretic (e.g. furosomide) may be used with caution.

Cough suppressants

Coughing is often an unpleasant symptom in many patients. However, coughing may in fact be of some advantage in COPD, especially if large amounts of sputum are produced. Cough suppressants are not known to provide any benefit in COPD, other than perhaps short-term use to control a particularly troublesome cough.

 FAQ

Will I always need to take drugs of some sort once COPD has been diagnosed?

Most people usually do need to take treatment for the rest of their lives.

Will my lung function return to normal if I take appropriate treatment?

Treatment usually improves lung function to some extent but does not usually return it to normal levels.

What are the similarities and differences between Symbicort and Seretide?

Both of these inhalers contain steroids and long-acting β_2-agonists and are used twice a day. Many clinical studies, involving large numbers of patients with COPD, have shown that both of these inhalers do improve lung function, reduce symptoms, and reduce the frequency of exacerbations.

The main difference is that they are delivered by different inhaler devices. On the whole, there is no clear consensus as to which one of the two drugs is more efficient than the other; whichever one is used should usually be a matter of patient preference. The inhaled steroid fluticasone is more potent than budesonide, while the long-acting β_2-agonist formoterol has a quicker onset of action than salmeterol.

7

Inhaler devices

> ## ➲ Key points
>
> ◆ A variety of different types of inhaler devices can be used to deliver different drugs to the lung.
>
> ◆ Some patients find difficulty in using hand-held inhaler devices properly. Even when used correctly, a substantial proportion of drug often is deposited in the mouth, throat, or vocal cords, with only a small amount reaching the lungs.
>
> ◆ Doctors, nurses, and pharmacists should ensure that patients use their inhaler correctly at the time of prescription.
>
> ◆ Nebulizers are no better at delivering drugs to the lung than a metered dose inhaler and spacer, if used correctly.

Inhaled drug treatment

The most effective drugs used in COPD are inhaled through the mouth. This makes intuitive sense, as this route of delivery means that drugs are directed to the problem area. Unfortunately, the major difficulty with most inhaled drugs is that only a small proportion actually reaches the lungs, as a considerable amount is often deposited in the mouth, throat, and vocal cords. This problem is made worse when there are problems co-ordinating inhaler devices, which may be more of an issue in older patients, in those with medical disorders affecting the hands or arms (such as arthritis), and in those who have difficulty in memorizing and retaining new information.

Prior to the introduction of inhaled treatment, it is crucial that patients:

◆ know what the drug is used for;

◆ know exactly when it should be used;

◆ are instructed on how to use the device correctly;

◆ are confident in using the particular device.

An assessment of inhaler technique should also be carried out at every available opportunity. This is important, as over time patients of all ages often become less able to use inhalers correctly.

Metered dose inhalers

One of the most common inhaler devices is a called a metered dose inhaler (MDI). To use an MDI correctly, patients should:

◆ remove the mouthpiece cover (if there is one) and shake the inhaler;

◆ breathe out fully (i.e. empty the lungs as completely as possible);

◆ put lips firmly around the mouthpiece;

◆ press *only once* with the inhaler in the mouth and at the same time breath inwards fully and deeply (i.e. fill the lungs as much as possible);

◆ hold breath for up to 10 s or for as long as is comfortable;

◆ breathe out normally;

◆ repeat these steps if a second puff is required;

◆ wipe the mouthpiece clean and replace its protective cover.

Many patients find difficulty in using MDIs, especially as it is often difficult to co-ordinate 'pressing' and 'sucking' at the same time. Other inhaler types have therefore been developed to help overcome this problem; many of these are called dry powder inhalers (DPIs). In general, whichever inhaler type the patient finds easy to use and feels confident in using is a reasonable way of deciding which one is best.

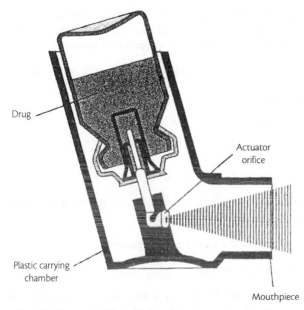

Drug

Actuator
orifice

Plastic carrying
chamber

Mouthpiece

Fig. 7.1 A drawing of a metered dose inhaler.

Use and maintenance of spacers

Some patients can develop a fungal infection of the mouth (called thrush) and complain of an alteration in the quality of their voice when using an MDI to deliver inhaled steroids to the lung. The risk of developing these problems can be minimized by:

◆ gargling with water after using the inhaler;

◆ rinsing the mouth after using the inhaler;

◆ brushing teeth after using the inhaler;

◆ using a spacer device.

A spacer is a large plastic container with an opening at either end: one opening is attached to the inhaler, and the other forms a mouthpiece. In general, they serve two functions. Firstly, they avoid problems in co-ordinating the timing of pressing the inhaler and 'sucking' inwards. Secondly, they slow down the speed of delivery of the aerosol into the mouth, which results in less drug being deposited in the mouth and throat. Different manufacturers make different sizes of spacers and inhalers, which should generally be used together. The following principles of use can be applied to most types of spacer:

◆ make sure the inhaler fits snugly into the end of the spacer device;

◆ breathe out fully;

◆ put lips around the mouthpiece;

◆ press the inhaler once;

◆ breathe inwards fully and deeply;

◆ hold breath for up to 10 s or for as long as is comfortable (alternatively take five normal breaths in and out);

◆ repeat these steps if a second puff is required;

◆ wipe the mouthpiece clean.

Spacers should generally be cleaned at least once a month with soapy water and be left to drip dry. They should be replaced every 6–12 months, depending on the manufacturer's recommendations.

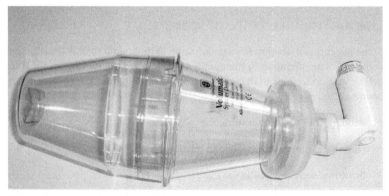

Fig. 7.2 A metered dose inhaler with spacer attached.

Other types of inhalers

An MDI used with a spacer device and a DPI are the most effective hand-held devices, providing they are used correctly. Despite being useful in delivering drugs to the lungs, the main drawbacks with spacers is the fact that many individuals feel they are bulky, less portable, and less convenient to use than DPIs. DPIs are designed to be breath-activated, which in turn overcomes the problem of co-ordination (when compared with using an MDI without a spacer). Several different types of breath-activated hand-held DPIs are available for use; commonly used types include Turbohalers, Accuhalers, and Easi-breathe inhalers.

Turbohalers

Turbohalers deliver drugs such as terbutaline, formoterol, budesonide, and formoterol plus budesonide in combination (Symbicort) to the lungs. To use a Turbohaler correctly, take the following steps:

◆ remove the outer cover and shake the inhaler;

◆ turn the base fully to the right and then back again until a click is heard;

◆ breathe out fully;

◆ put lips around the mouthpiece and breathe inwards fully and deeply;

◆ hold breath for up to 10 s or for as long as is comfortable;

◆ repeat these steps if a second puff is required;

◆ wipe the mouthpiece clean and replace the outer cover.

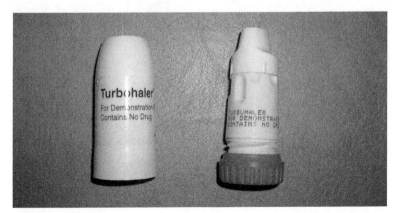

Fig. 7.3 A Turbohaler.

Accuhalers

Accuhalers deliver drugs such as salbutamol, salmeterol, fluticasone, and salmeterol plus fluticasone in combination (Seretide) to the lungs. To use an Accuhaler correctly, take the following steps:

♦ open the device by pressing down on the thumb rest;

♦ click the lever down as far as possible;

♦ breathe out fully;

♦ put lips around the mouthpiece and ensure a good seal;

♦ breathe inwards fully and deeply;

♦ hold breath for up to 10 s or for as long as is comfortable;

♦ wipe the mouthpiece clean and close the device.

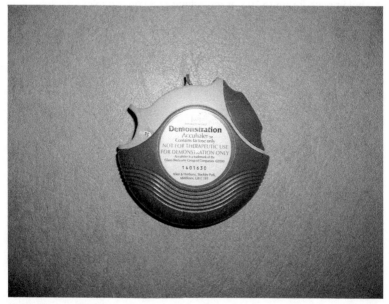

Fig. 7.4 An Accuhaler.

Easi-breathe inhalers

Easi-breathe inhalers deliver drugs such as salbutamol and beclomethasone to the lungs. To use an Easi-breathe inhaler correctly, take the following steps:

♦ shake the inhaler;

♦ open the cap covering the mouthpiece;

♦ breathe out fully;

♦ put lips around the mouthpiece and ensure a good seal (take care not to block the air holes);

♦ breathe inwards fully and deeply;

♦ hold breath for up to 10 s or for as long as is comfortable;

♦ repeat these steps if a second puff is required;

♦ wipe the mouthpiece clean and put the cap back over the mouthpiece.

Handihaler

The Handihaler delivers tiotropium (Spireva) to the lungs. To use a Handihaler correctly, take the following steps:

♦ open the outer lid and inner white mouthpiece;

♦ place a capsule into the inner basket;

♦ press the button at the side of the inhaler once (this pierces the capsule);

♦ breathe out fully;

♦ put lips around the mouthpiece and ensure a good seal;

♦ breathe inwards fully and deeply;

♦ hold breath for up to 10 s or for as long as is comfortable;

♦ repeating these steps is often useful to ensure that most of the drug from within the capsule is used;

♦ wipe the mouthpiece clean and place the cap back over the mouthpiece.

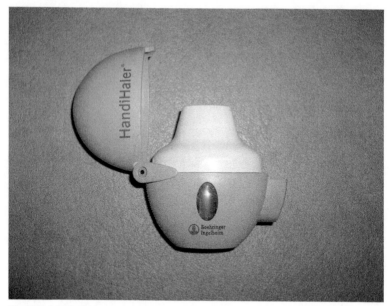

Fig. 7.5 A Handihaler.

 Patient's perspective

Mr Q, aged 62

Eighteen months on from being diagnosed with COPD, quitting smoking, and with the help of inhaled medication, my day-to-day life is virtually untouched by COPD. I am unaware of the presence of the condition, except on those occasions when I push myself too hard physically. Visits to my GP for antibiotics have ceased, there has never been a requirement for me to attend hospital out-patient clinics (other than once to see a chest specialist); admissions to hospital have not been necessary. As I am now retired, any stresses and strains from employment have been removed from the equation.

My family and I were concerned for my future when COPD was diagnosed. However, 18 months later those concerns have evaporated as the benefits of quitting smoking have taken effect, along with the benefits of medication, and reassurance and advice provided by nursing and medical staff.

Tools to help you use inhaler devices

If you have arthritis or any other painful condition affecting your hands, a device called a Haleraid or Turboaid may be useful. These devices fit onto some types of inhalers and allow you to release the drug by applying pressure with the palm of your hand. Many patients find this far easier to do than using some devices.

Nebulizers

Nebulizers are small, relatively portable machines, which are powered from the electric mains or even from a car lighter. They are driven by compressed air or oxygen and create a mist of drug particles, which in turn is inhaled by the patient via a face mask or mouthpiece.

Nebulizers tend to be used during an exacerbation of COPD, either at home, in an ambulance, or in hospital. Some patients with more advanced COPD use a nebulizer at home on a regular or intermittent basis. However, it is important to point out that using a nebulizer is probably as effective as using an MDI plus spacer correctly. Furthermore, despite delivering far higher doses than inhalers, nebulizers tend to be inefficient, as most of the aerosol mist containing the drug is lost to the atmosphere. Using a nebulizer can take as long as 10–20 min, while using an inhaler takes only a fraction of this time. Nebulizers are also expensive and require servicing from time to time.

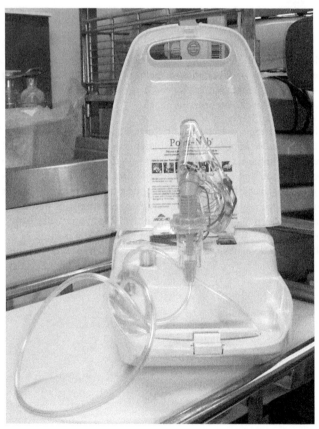

Fig. 7.6 A nebulizer.

FAQ

What is the best inhaler device for me?

This is impossible to answer as individuals differ greatly. In general, whatever inhaler you find easiest to use is probably the best one for you. Ideally, your nurse or pharmacist should show you the different types of inhaler and discuss which one you would prefer to use.

Can I take a tablet instead of an inhaler?

Unfortunately not. Inhalers are the best way by which to deliver the best drugs for COPD into your lungs.

Should I have a nebulizer once COPD has been diagnosed?

No. Patients often feel a nebulizer is better than inhalers at delivering drugs to them, although this is not backed up by good scientific evidence. It should usually be as a last resort that a nebulizer is prescribed or when a patient is unable to use inhaler devices.

8

Oxygen and COPD

⮑ Key points

♦ You are usually given oxygen if you are admitted to hospital with an exacerbation of COPD; this is usually delivered by way of a face mask or nasal cannula.

♦ 'Short burst' oxygen therapy (using oxygen from a cylinder for short periods of time at home) is thought to be of little benefit in relieving symptoms. However, it may occasionally be considered if you have severe, persistent, and disabling symptoms despite all other treatments.

♦ A minority of patients with more severe COPD, with low oxygen levels, and who have stopped smoking, may benefit from oxygen at home. This should be delivered through a machine called an oxygen concentrator and used for at least 15 h each day.

♦ Patients with more advanced COPD should ideally have oxygen levels checked before arranging an aircraft flight. If oxygen levels are sufficiently low, in-flight oxygen may need to be organized for the duration of the flight.

The atmospheric air at ground level, which we all breathe, is made up of around 21% oxygen, 78% nitrogen, and a small quantity of other gases. However, oxygen is considered a drug when prescribed to patients with COPD. This is largely because inappropriate use of oxygen may cause worsening of a patient's clinical condition and therefore consideration always needs to be given before supplemental oxygen is given either in hospital or at home.

Oxygen during an exacerbation

Oxygen should be given to patients with low oxygen levels in the blood who have an exacerbation of COPD and are admitted to hospital. It is usually delivered by means of a face mask held in place around the head with an elastic strap; it may also be given through nasal cannulae or 'prongs'. To check that an adequate amount of oxygen is being given, the oxygen level will often be monitored by a small machine called a pulse oximeter. In order to check that carbon dioxide levels are not rising (which can sometimes happen if too much oxygen is administered), a blood test (called an arterial blood gas) may be taken from time to time usually from an artery at the wrist. As clinical condition improves, the oxygen concentration given through the face mask is usually decreased gradually and discontinued.

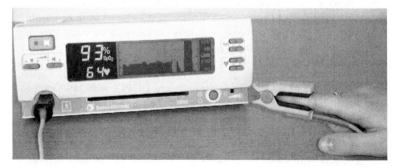

Fig. 8.1 A pulse oximeter.

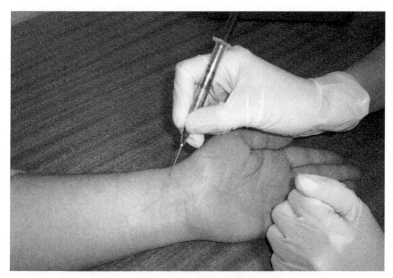

Fig. 8.2 Patient having an arterial blood gas measurement taken from the wrist.

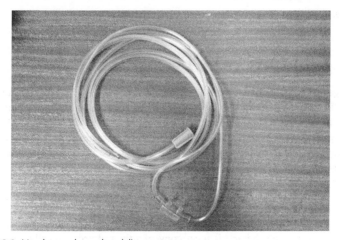

Fig. 8.3 Nasal cannula used to deliver oxygen.

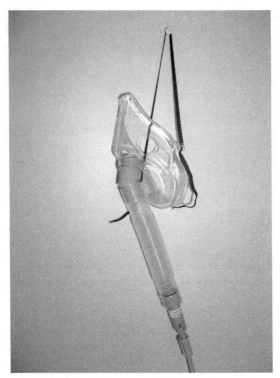

Fig. 8.4 Face mask used to deliver oxygen.

Long-term oxygen therapy

Oxygen at home is usually only considered in patients with fairly advanced COPD who have completely given up smoking for at least 3 months. Current guidelines issued to doctors indicate that if a patient has sufficiently low levels of oxygen in their blood, long-term oxygen therapy at home provides benefit, mainly in terms of living longer. For this benefit to be achieved, oxygen needs to be used for at least 15 h over a 24-h period. Patients are often initially discouraged at the thought of using oxygen for this length of time, although using it overnight while sleeping may make up a significant proportion of the recommended 15 h a day.

Long-term oxygen therapy is most conveniently and economically given by a machine called a concentrator; this is roughly the size of a small fridge.

This machine removes nitrogen from the atmosphere and produces oxygen-enriched air to breathe. Oxygen is most conveniently delivered via nasal cannulae, although some patients—especially those who are troubled with drying and crusting of the inside of the nose—may prefer a face mask.

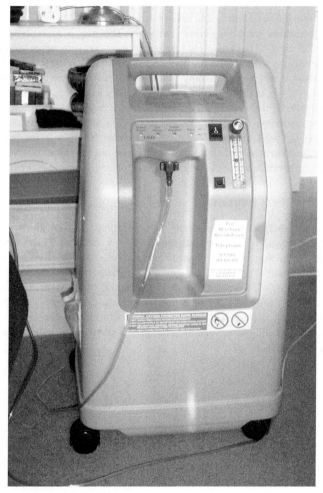

Fig. 8.5 An oxygen concentrator.

To determine whether long-term oxygen therapy is indicated or not, the doctor or nurse needs firstly to check blood oxygen level using a pulse oximeter. Depending on this result, a formal assessment of the amount of oxygen in the patient's actual blood may need to be carried out. This involves taking a sample of blood from an artery, usually at the wrist.

'Short burst' oxygen

Despite maximum non-drug and drug treatment for COPD, some patients will remain breathless when they exert themselves. This may occur without a significant fall in blood oxygen levels. Oxygen cylinders are sometimes prescribed to these patients for use 'if and when' they are particularly breathless—this is called 'short burst' oxygen therapy. Clinical studies have generally not shown that using oxygen in this way is of any great benefit; as a result, it is not usually recommended. Furthermore, oxygen cylinders are bulky and difficult to transport, are expensive, and generally only last for up to 8 h depending on how often they are used and the flow rate. Nevertheless, 'short burst' oxygen may be considered in a very small minority of patients with episodes of severe and debilitating breathlessness not relieved by any other treatments.

Ambulatory oxygen

Some patients receiving long-term oxygen therapy can be given a small cylinder of oxygen to carry around with them in a backpack. This means that they can receive a continual flow of oxygen while outside their home and is called ambulatory oxygen. This method of delivering oxygen is of some use in a number of patients, although it is limited by the fact that some cylinders only last for up to 4 h with a low flow rate and even less with a higher flow rate. In the future, small, lightweight cylinders, oxygen-conserving devices, and portable liquid oxygen systems may become more widely available within the UK.

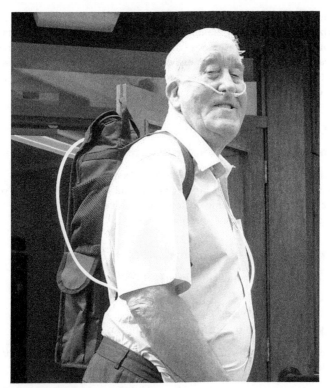

Fig. 8.6 A patient using ambulatory oxygen.

Air travel

An increasing number of individuals at the extremes of age and with a variety of medical illnesses such as COPD are choosing to fly in aircraft. Even in healthy individuals, oxygen levels fall slightly when at altitude. If oxygen levels are already low because of COPD, then they may fall to a potentially worrying levels during a flight.

In view of this, the oxygen level while breathing room air should ideally be measured using a pulse oximeter before airline flights are booked—especially in those with more advanced COPD. Doing so helps determine whether oxygen during the flight is required or not. If oxygen is needed, inform the relevant airline when booking and be aware that some airlines charge for this service.

Individuals with more advanced disease should also consider whether oxygen (and even a wheelchair) on the ground and while changing flights will be required. Carry all necessary inhalers on board the flight as hand luggage; nebulizers may be used at the discretion of the cabin crew. It is important to take out the necessary insurance when travelling abroad in case emergency medical assistance is required. Patients may also find it useful and reassuring to have a supply of antibiotics and steroids to take with them on holiday to use in the event of an exacerbation of COPD.

 FAQ

Can I be given oxygen for use at home if I continue to smoke?

This is generally not advised due to the risks of starting a fire. If oxygen has already been installed in your house, and it is discovered that you have started smoking, some doctors may feel it necessary to remove the oxygen concentrator from your house.

Is there a chance of becoming addicted to oxygen?

No, oxygen is not an addictive drug.

If I have been advised to use oxygen on a long-term basis, why do I need to use it for at least 15 h a day?

Several clinical studies have shown *no* long-term benefit if oxygen is used for less than 15 h each day.

Will I become housebound if oxygen is given to me all the time at home?

No, this is far from the intention. Keeping as active as possible is one of the best things that you can do.

Can I drive my car while using oxygen?

The answer here is yes. However, you should inform your insurance company.

Can I go to the shops, cinema, pub, or restaurant if I use ambulatory oxygen?

Yes. However, make sure you have sufficient oxygen in your cylinder and avoid potential sources of ignition.

9

Episodes of worsening symptoms (exacerbations)

➲ Key points

♦ Most patients with COPD will experience a worsening of symptoms (called an exacerbation) at some time; these should be treated promptly.

♦ Most exacerbations can be successfully managed at home with short courses of steroid tablets and antibiotics, and increased use of reliever inhalers.

♦ If admitted to hospital, patients will probably receive oxygen, high-dose inhaled bronchodilators (drugs to open up the airways) and a short course of steroid tablets and antibiotics.

♦ A minority of patients with more severe exacerbations may require help to breathe using a machine called a ventilator.

♦ Once an exacerbation of COPD has settled, patients should be followed-up by their doctor or nurse.

Once diagnosed with COPD, patients may, from time to time, experience a fairly abrupt worsening of symptoms, which requires them to seek advice and assistance from a doctor or nurse. This is termed an exacerbation. Exacerbations of COPD account for around 10% of all admissions to hospital wards in the UK, which amounts to over 100 000 admissions each year. This happens more commonly in winter months and in those with more advanced disease and increasing age. Most patients are treated safely and successfully outside hospital in their own home. The precise cause of an exacerbation of COPD is often uncertain, but different viruses, bacteria, or pollutants in the atmosphere are often thought to be responsible.

Features of an exacerbation include increased breathlessness, cough, wheeze, and chest tightness, and a greater volume of sputum production and darkening of its colour. Other features that may be present include a feeling of general ill health, fever, a reduction in the distance that can easily be walked, a blue discoloration around the lips, fluid retention, and, occasionally, confusion; patients may only have a few, rather than all, of these symptoms. Patients do not normally cough up blood or complain of severe chest pain during an exacerbation of COPD; if this occurs, hospital admission is usually necessary.

 Patient's perspective

Mr M, aged 52

Having a bath or a shower can leave me very drained. Getting dressed in the morning can sometimes take up to 20 minutes as I need to take a seat to catch my breath in between putting on clothes. First thing in the morning, it takes quite a while to get going; it's like your lungs are not awake and then they start to function better. When walking down the street I tend to walk a little, and then stop for a rest before I get too breathless. This enables me to be more in control of my breathing rather than getting so out of breath that I begin to panic. If you do lose control of your breathing on exertion, it can be a very scary experience. Having a bad chest infection can also be a scary time. So you have to try and avoid them if you can by looking after yourself, like wrapping up in cold weather and avoiding contact with anyone with colds or the flu.

Whenever I am going anywhere I have not been before, I try to do a bit of forward planning. For example, I try to find out things like can I get parked? How far will I have to walk? Are there stairs or a lift? You sometimes get breathless doing the simplest of tasks, as how you are feeling varies from day to day. Some days you just feel totally exhausted. Your confidence also takes a bit of a knock.

Sleeping is also a problem; I find it difficult to get to sleep, wake up after a short while, and never seem to get a good solid sleep. You have to keep motivated and get out and about, and not just sit at home, as the more you try and do the better you will feel in mind as well as body. You really have to try and live your life as normal as possible.

Work, family, and the future

I was struggling to cope at work and started to have more time off due to my condition, but am pleased to say my employers were very good and allowed me to go part-time. At work, I still struggle at times and I do get anxious and embarrassed if I have difficulty catching my breath, although my colleagues are very helpful and always willing to lend a hand. My family are all very supportive and my wife looks after me very well. I am optimistic about the future.

Should I be treated in hospital or at home?

You should report symptoms of an exacerbation of COPD to your GP at an early stage. This is very important, since early and prompt treatment results in a quicker recovery. Moreover, patients who fail to report worsening symptoms and receive treatment promptly have a greater risk of being admitted to hospital.

The vast majority of patients with an exacerbation of COPD can be safely and effectively treated at home. However, if any of the following features are present, it may mean that they would be better managed in hospital:

- no-one else at home;

- unable to manage at home;

- no family or friends nearby available to help if necessary;

- difficulty walking around the house or confined to bed;

- other medical illnesses (e.g. heart disease, kidney disease, or diabetes);

- uncertainty as to whether an exacerbation of COPD is the diagnosis;

- severe breathlessness, wheeze, or chest tightness;

- a blue discoloration around the mouth;

- worsening ankle swelling;

- chest pain;

- coughing up blood;

- confusion;

- low oxygen levels;

- already receiving long-term oxygen at home.

Home treatment

If the decision has been made to manage a patient's exacerbation at home, a 7–14-day course of steroid tablets (usually prednisolone) and oral antibiotics for up to 7 days will usually be prescribed. A 'reliever' inhaler should be used as often as necessary and use of the 'preventer' inhaler should be continued. Even if the initial decision is that for treatment at home, admission to hospital may take place at a later stage, if the condition or circumstances change.

Hospital treatment

If admitted to hospital, patients will initially be assessed by a doctor and nurse. As well as in-depth details regarding current symptoms, patients will also be asked a series of questions regarding any other medical problems they may have, drugs and inhalers that they take (these should be brought in with the patient), social circumstances, occupation, mobility, presence of allergies, family history of any medical disorders, and smoking status.

The doctor or nurse should then ask permission to carry out an examination. If the patient agrees, they will probably conduct a full examination paying particular attention to the chest and heart. During this process, temperature, pulse rate, breathing rate, blood pressure, and oxygen level will be measured. There will then probably be a variety of investigations such as blood tests (usually at least blood count, kidney function, and sugar level), a heart tracing (ECG), and a chest X-ray. If coughing up sputum, this should also be sent off to the laboratory to help determine if a particular bacterium is responsible for the exacerbation (although the result may take several days to come back). This may help decide which antibiotics should be given. If the decision is made to keep the patient in hospital, some or most of the following treatments may be given.

Oxygen

Many patients with an exacerbation of COPD have low oxygen levels. To deal with this, oxygen is usually given via a face mask or nasal cannula. To ensure sufficient oxygen is being given and that waste gas (carbon dioxide) levels are not rising, further blood tests (called arterial blood gases) may be taken—usually from one of the arteries at the wrist—from time to time (Fig 8.2). Oxygen levels may also be monitored (either all the time or from time to time) by a pulse oximeter; this involves inserting a finger into a probe, which is attached to a small machine by the bedside (Fig 8.1).

Bronchodilators

Drugs to open up the airways—called bronchodilators—will also be given. These drugs act within several minutes to relieve breathlessness. Bronchodilators may be given through a nebulizer or hand-held inhaler with a spacer attached. The most common types of bronchodilators are called salbutamol and ipratropium. They can be given alone or in combination. These drugs last up to 6 h and are therefore usually given several times on a regular basis throughout a 24-h period. The main side-effects of these types of drugs are palpitations (an awareness of a fast heart beat) and tremor of the hands.

Steroids

Steroid tablets (most commonly prednisolone) will also usually be given for an exacerbation. The length of the course varies from person to person, but should usually be 7–14 days. If the patient is very ill or has swallowing difficulties, steroids may be given straight into a vein through a plastic cannula (drip) situated in the back of the hand or forearm. A single short course of steroid tablets is not usually associated with major side-effects, but they may cause a temporary increase in appetite, a general sense of well-being, increased energy levels, and some weight gain. Patients who are given repeated short courses of steroid tablets for frequent exacerbations may also run into the problems encountered by those receiving them every day on a long-term basis (see Chapter 6).

Antibiotics

Antibiotics may be given to treat an exacerbation of COPD; they are most effective if increased breathlessness and increased sputum volume with darkening of its colour are experienced. However, it is important to remember that the majority of respiratory tract infections are caused by viruses, which do not respond to antibiotics. Over the years, widespread antibiotic use has been associated with the emergence of MRSA (a bacterium that does not respond to conventional antibiotics) and *Clostridium difficile* (a bacterium in the bowel that causes fever, bloody diarrhoea, and abdominal pain). Doctors or nurses may decide not to prescribe antibiotics, especially if the exacerbation is mild.

However, if there is no improvement and sputum remains discoloured, antibiotics may then need to be started.

Antibiotics are usually given by mouth, although they may be given straight into a vein through a plastic cannula in more severe exacerbations, or if there are swallowing difficulties. It is important that medical and nursing staff are informed if the patient is allergic to penicillin, as a form of penicillin (such as amoxycillin or co-amoxiclav) is the most commonly used antibiotic. If a patient is allergic to penicillin, an antibiotic called clarithromycin or erythromycin may be given. Common side-effects of most antibiotics include nausea, vomiting, and diarrhoea; the patient should let their doctor or nurse know if any of these features are severe or prolonged. The choice of antibiotic may alter during a stay in hospital, since results from sputum tests may indicate that a different antibiotic may be more effective. Antibiotics are usually given for up to a week.

Aminophylline

In more severe exacerbations that do not respond to the measures above, a drug called aminophylline may be given; this can have some benefit in opening up (dilating) the airways even further. Aminophylline can only be given through a plastic cannula directly into a vein. Doctors are prescribing it less frequently nowadays, as there are more effective alternatives; many scientific studies have also suggested that it may not be terribly effective. Moreover, many individuals find themselves unable to tolerate this drug as it often causes nausea, vomiting, and an increased heart rate resulting in uncomfortable 'palpitations'. To keep a check on the heart rate, patients are often attached to a monitor, by means of sticky electrodes placed on the chest, while this drug is given. It is usually only prescribed for several days, but stopped earlier if side-effects occur.

Other treatments

Patients may easily become dehydrated with a severe and prolonged exacerbation of COPD; fluids containing salt and water (a saline drip) may therefore be given directly into a vein. Fluids through a drip are usually stopped once dehydration has been corrected and the patient is able to eat and drink normally. If the patient remains at home during an exacerbation, it is important that they drink plenty of clear fluids.

Most people admitted to hospital are not as mobile as they have been, which means an increased risk of developing a clot (deep venous thrombosis or 'DVT') within the veins of the leg. If this happens, the clot can spread into the lung (and cause a pulmonary embolism), which further complicates respiratory difficulties. To help prevent this, compression stockings or daily injections into the skin of a blood-thinning drug (heparin) should usually be given. These measures are stopped once patients are mobile.

Ventilation

Some patients with more severe exacerbations have difficulty exhaling the waste gas carbon dioxide and inhaling sufficient quantities of oxygen. As a result of the extra work of breathing, they can also become tired and develop weakness of the chest muscles; this all may cause levels of oxygen to fall and carbon dioxide to rise. In these circumstances, artificial help with breathing using a machine (ventilator) may be needed. Two main types of assisted breathing are possible and are called non-invasive ventilation and invasive ventilation.

 FAQ

How many exacerbations should I expect to have each year?

This is very variable and impossible to predict with any degree of certainty, as some people have several exacerbations while others may have none at all. The important thing is that exacerbations are treated promptly, as doing so has been shown in clinical studies to reduce the time taken to recover.

Can I be involved in making decisions as to whether I am considered for artificial means to help me breathe (ventilation)?

Yes. Nowadays, it is often preferable to discuss with doctors and nurses whether you would like to be ventilated using either invasive or non-invasive ventilation. Once you have recovered from an exacerbation, it is also very useful to comment whether you would wish to be ventilated in the future. It may be useful to discuss these decisions with next of kin, other close family member, doctors, and nurses.

Non-invasive ventilation

Non-invasive ventilation is widely used in most hospitals, and is the most common form of ventilation in COPD. It involves connecting a patient to a portable bedside ventilator by means of plastic tubing and a close fitting face or nose mask, attached by a band around the head. The mask can be removed easily, which means that the patient can talk, eat, drink, and receive nebulized and oral medication without difficulty. This form of treatment is very successful and may be necessary for only a few hours or up to several days. It may also be stopped for short periods of time. Non-invasive ventilation is usually continued until blood gas levels have improved (oxygen levels higher and carbon dioxide levels lower) and the patient is feeling more comfortable and less breathless. Arterial blood gases are usually performed on a fairly regular basis while using the non-invasive ventilator.

Non-invasive ventilation has greatly improved the management of patients with more severe exacerbations of COPD, although at times it should be avoided. For example, it is not recommended if patients have persistent vomiting, facial burns, a reduced conscious level, or if individuals with advanced severe disease are thought to be near death.

 FAQ

If I am started on non-invasive ventilation, how long will I require it for?

This varies widely between different people. In some, only a few hours of treatment are necessary, but in others several days of non-invasive ventilation are required.

How is non-invasive ventilation different from being given oxygen through a mask?

Non-invasive ventilation provides both a flow of oxygen into your lungs and a form of 'pressure support'. This pressure support helps to keep your airways open and does some of the work of your breathing muscles when you become tired.

Is non-invasive ventilation uncomfortable?

Not really. Most patients tolerate non-invasive ventilation without too much difficulty. Before being started on it, it is useful to hold the mask in your own hands and to hold it over your face, to give you a feeling of what is feels like prior to having it strapped around your head. Pressure settings on the non-invasive ventilator are also usually started fairly low to enable you to 'get used to' the machine and the feeling of air being blown in to your lungs; as time goes on, the pressures are often gradually increased providing you feel comfortable. If non-invasive ventilation is used for a prolonged period, you may get a break in the skin or 'sore' developing across the bridge of your nose; this can usually be rectified by using different techniques.

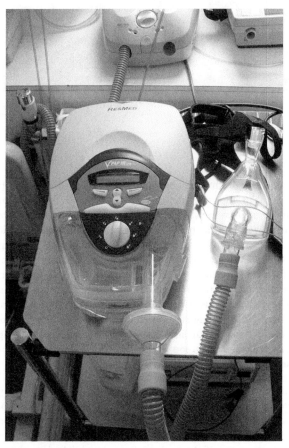

Fig. 9.1 A non-invasive ventilator.

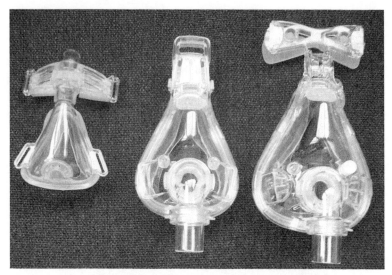

Fig. 9.2 A variety of nasal or full face masks can be used to deliver non-invasive ventilation.

Invasive ventilation

In some patients, non-invasive ventilation may be unavailable, inappropriate, or unsuccessful in improving the clinical condition. In these circumstances, patients are sometimes transferred to the intensive care unit for more invasive ventilation. This means that patients will be sedated (made unconscious) with anaesthetic drugs and have a plastic tube inserted into their windpipe (trachea) through their mouth. This tube will then be connected to a ventilator by means of further plastic tubing. This will continue, with the ventilator allowing the patient to gradually take over the work of breathing, until it is no longer needed. This form of invasive ventilation may be inappropriate at times. For example, some patients may have stated beforehand that they do not wish to be considered for this treatment, while others may have pre-existing COPD, or other medical conditions, too severe for invasive ventilation to be considered of benefit.

If a patient is very unwell and thought to require assisted breathing with an invasive ventilator for a more prolonged period of time, doctors may create something called a tracheostomy in the neck. This means that, instead of the plastic tube being inserted into the mouth, it will be put through a small cut made in the front of the neck and passed straight into the windpipe.

This tube is attached by further plastic tubing to the ventilator. Doing this helps to reduce the amount of time that the patient needs to be attached to the ventilator. Having a tracheostomy inserted is painless, as the patient is made unconscious with anaesthetic drugs at the time. After the patient has recovered sufficiently, the tracheostomy is easily removed and the hole created in the neck heals up and closes over within a few weeks.

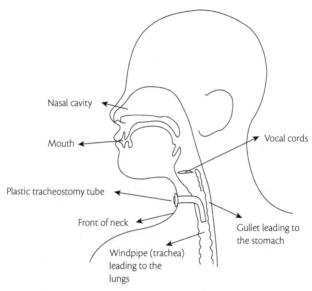

Fig. 9.3 Diagrammatic 'side-on view' of a tracheostomy.

Discharge home

'Hospital at home' or 'assisted discharge' schemes for patients with mild exacerbations of COPD are becoming more widespread in the UK. These schemes enable patients to be safely discharged back home earlier than would normally be anticipated, with nursing support and treatment provided at home. This allows patients to recuperate and be assessed on a frequent basis at home where they can be offered appropriate advice and reassurance, where necessary. Depending on the hospital, patients may initially be assessed in an out-patient department without reaching a ward and sent home with the necessary treatment. In other hospitals, they may be admitted to a ward for a short period of time (perhaps 24–48 h) before being discharged home. These schemes also mean that patients are not kept in hospital unnecessarily, which results in potential financial savings without compromising their care, safety, satisfaction, or outcome. It also means that there is less chance of patients catching further infections while in hospital. Experience also indicates that patients prefer to be kept at home, if possible, during an exacerbation of COPD, as long as appropriate treatment, reassurance, and follow-up are provided.

Follow-up

Once recovery from an exacerbation has taken place, many hospitals arrange to follow-up patients at an out-patient clinic 4–6 weeks after discharge. Some form of follow-up should also be arranged by the GP, if an exacerbation was treated at home. This gives an opportunity to provide further education, and allows the doctor or nurse to consider changing treatment, to check inhaler technique, vaccination status, oxygen levels, and lung function, and to re-assess smoking status, where necessary.

End-of-life issues

Dying and death are inevitable and can be considered to be nature's way of ensuring that the cycle of human life continues. Some patients with COPD die because of it, others die of other problems such as heart disease, which commonly co-exists with it, while many others die in their sleep or merely due to old age. In some patients with COPD who are considered to be dying (whether at home or in hospital), it may clearly be inappropriate to initiate aggressive treatment, such as non-invasive ventilation or drugs given through drips. Moreover, following an initial period of active management when the prognosis is uncertain, it may become clear that treatment is ineffective and it is appropriate to consider its withdrawal. This should usually be decided following discussion with patients themselves (if possible) and their families. In these circumstances, the goal then becomes to ensure that symptoms are adequately assessed and treated, and that death occurs naturally and peacefully. This may mean that drugs that reduce discomfort, pain, anxiety, and the sensation of breathlessness are given. Examples of these include oxygen, morphine-based drugs, a class of drugs called benzodiazepines, which include diazepam, lorazepam, and midazolam, and drugs to dry up airway secretions. It is also important to ensure that patients are turned in bed (when indicated), that oral and personal hygiene are maintained, dignity is preserved, and over-all care is adequately provided, whether at home or in hospital. Some patients may request a member of the clergy to be present.

Advanced directives

Over the past few years, advanced directives have become more widespread. These are legal documents and mean that, if circumstances arise such that a patient is unable to consent to treatment—and that treatment is likely to be useless—the patient would not wish medical intervention to support or sustain life of dubious quality. In advanced COPD, this may refer to artificial ventilation, cardiopulmonary resuscitation (trying to restart the heart if it were to stop beating), fluids given through a drip, and artificial feeding. Some people might regard this as a way of ensuring that death occurs in a dignified manner without the fear of interventions being initiated, which are exceedingly unlikely to be successful or prolong life. Advanced directives cannot be over-ruled by doctors, family, and friends provided that they are correctly and legally drawn up, although they can be changed or withdrawn at any time if the individual is mentally competent to do so. Doctors, nurses, family, and next of kin should know that such a document exists and where it is kept; it may be appropriate and useful to have a copy filed in the patient's case notes. It is usually advisable to have a solicitor involved in the formation of an advanced directive and have it clearly dated and signed by witnesses.

 FAQ

Will it hurt if I die from COPD?

Doctors and nurses are trained to identify discomfort in people who are dying and will do their utmost to avoid patients experiencing unpleasant and distressing breathlessness, coughing, anxiety, or pain. This can usually be easily achieved with different types of drugs, which can be swallowed or injected.

If I am dying from COPD, will doctors and nurses be less inclined to treat my symptoms efficiently?

Absolutely not. You should receive the same level of care whether you have a mild, moderate, severe, or life-threatening exacerbation of COPD. Patients who are thought to be dying will also receive a similar high level of care and attention.

Appendix 1

Glossary of drugs

Most drugs have a common (generic) name and a name given to it by the manufacturer (brand name); the name given to a particular drug (or inhaler device) may even be different depending in which country you live! This may easily result in confusion, as you may be familiar with the generic name of a drug but be unfamiliar with its alternative brand name. Below is a short glossary of the drugs most commonly used in COPD, which highlights their generic name, drug company (brand) name, main mode of action, use, and frequency of use.

Generic name: formoterol

Brand (Drug Company) name: Oxis, Foradil, Atimos

Main mode of action: opens the airway for a prolonged period of time

Use: prevention of symptoms and exacerbations

Frequency of use: twice a day

Generic name: formoterol and budesonide (combined in a single inhaler)

Brand (Drug Company) name: Symbicort (Oxis and Pulmicort)

Main mode of action: opens the airway for a prolonged period of time and reduces inflammation

Use: prevention of symptoms and reduction in exacerbations

Frequency of use: twice a day

Generic name: ipratropium

Brand (Drug Company) name: Atrovent

Main mode of action: opens the airway

Use: rapid relief of symptoms

Frequency of use: on an as-required basis or 3–4 times a day

Generic name: ipratropium and salbutamol (used in nebules for a nebulizer)

Brand (Drug Company) name: Combivent

Main mode of action: opens the airway

Use: rapid relief of symptoms

Frequency of use: on an as-required basis or 3–4 times a day

Generic name: prednisolone

Brand (Drug Company) name: prednisolone

Main mode of action: reduces inflammation

Use: treatment of exacerbations or occasionally for long-term use in patients with advanced disease

Frequency of use: usually once a day

Generic name: salbutamol

Brand (Drug Company) name: Ventolin, Salamol, Airomir, Asmasal

Main mode of action: opens the airway

Use: rapid relief of symptoms

Frequency of use: on an as-required basis

Generic name: salmeterol

Brand (Drug Company) name: Serevent

Main mode of action: opens the airway for a prolonged period of time

Use: prevention of symptoms and exacerbations

Frequency of use: twice a day

Generic name: salmeterol and fluticasone (combined in a single inhaler)

Brand (Drug Company) name: Seretide (Serevent and Flixotide)

Main mode of action: opens the airway for a prolonged period of time and reduces inflammation

Use: prevention of symptoms and reduction in exacerbations

Frequency of use: twice a day

Generic name: terbutaline

Brand (Drug Company) name: Bricanyl

Main mode of action: opens the airway

Use: rapid relief of symptoms

Frequency of use: on an as-required basis

Generic name: theophylline

Brand (Drug Company) name: Uniphyllin, Nuelin, Slo-Phyllin

Main mode of action: opens the airway

Use: prevention of symptoms

Frequency of use: once or twice a day depending on the manufacturer's recommendations

Generic name: tiotropium

Brand (Drug Company) name: Spiriva

Main mode of action: opens the airway for a prolonged period of time

Use: prevention of symptoms and exacerbations

Frequency of use: once a day

Appendix 2

Further information

You may have found out other information about COPD from a variety of sources such as television, radio, books, and magazines. More recently, many individuals of all ages have gained access to the world wide web. Although this is an invaluable source of information, some websites may contain inaccurate or at worst misleading information. It is also important to be aware that some treatments advertised on the internet have not been rigorously investigated in clinical trials and may not be endorsed by the medical, nursing, or pharmacy professions. It is therefore imperative that any issues arising from access to the internet, involving even minor treatment changes, are discussed fully with your doctor, nurse, or pharmacist.

Websites providing further information regarding COPD and its management

www.chss.org.uk

www.brit-thoracic.org.uk

www.lunguk.org

www.laia.ac.uk

www.bnf.org

Websites providing further information on smoking cessation

www.canstopsmoking.com

www.quit.org.uk

www.givingupsmoking.co.uk

www.ash.org.uk

Websites providing further information on holidays, benefits, and mobility aids

www.holidaycare.org.uk

www.motability.co.uk

www.dwp.giv.uk.lifeevent/benefits

Index